DANVILLE PUBLIC LIBRARY

3 1205 00

C0-AZE-428

WITHDRAWN

636.089 DUN
Duncan, Jane Caryl.
Careers in veterinary
medicine

| | DATE DUE | | |
|---|---|---|---|
| OCT 0 6 2014 | | | |
| | | | |
| | | | |
| | | | |
| | | | |
| | | | |
| | | | |
| | | | |
| | | | |
| | | | |

# CAREERS IN VETERINARY MEDICINE

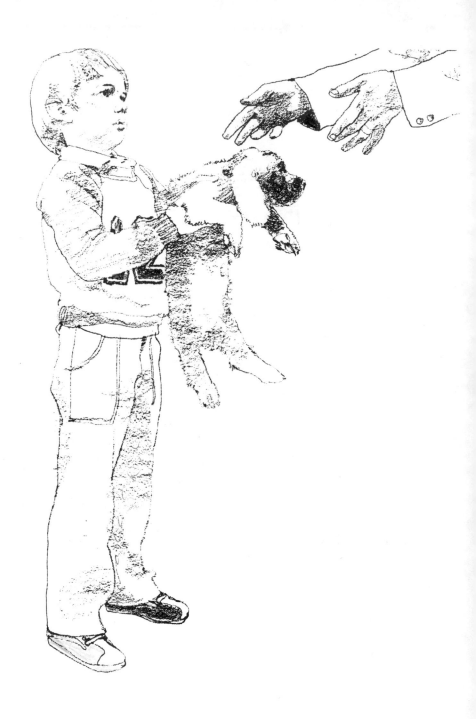

# CAREERS IN VETERINARY MEDICINE

*By*

Jane Caryl Duncan, D.V.M.

THE ROSEN PUBLISHING GROUP, Inc.

New York

Published in 1988 by The Rosen Publishing Group, Inc.
29 East 21st Street, New York, NY 10010

*Copyright 1988 by Jane Caryl Duncan*

All rights reserved. No part of this book may be
reproduced in any form without permission in writing
from the publisher, except by a reviewer.

*First Edition*

LIBRARY OF CONGRESS
Library of Congress Cataloging-in-Publication Data

Duncan, Jane Caryl.
    Careers in veterinary medicine / by Jane Caryl Duncan.
— 1st ed.
        p.   cm. — (Careers in depth)
    Bibliography index.
    Summary: Discusses various opportunities in the field of
veterinary medicine and the education and training necessary
for a career.
    ISBN 0-8239-0804-6:  $9.97
        1. Veterinary medicine—Vocational guidance.      [1.
Veterinary medicine—Vocational guidance.   2. Vocational
guidance.]   I. Title.
    II. Series.
    [DNLM: 1. Veterinary Medicine.   SF 745 D911c]
SF756.28.D86   1988
636.089'023'73—dc19
DNLM/DLC
for Library of Congress                                   88-4672
                                                              CIP
                                                              AC

*Manufactured in the United States of America*

636.089
DUN
cop. 1

# About the Author

Jane Caryl Duncan received her Bachelor of Science degree in Biology, summa cum laude, from the College of St. Francis in Joliet, Illinois, in 1975. Four years later she fulfilled her lifelong dream of becoming a veterinarian by obtaining her Doctor of Veterinary Medicine degree from the University of Illinois.

After being employed for one year in northern Indiana as a clinical veterinarian for pets, horses, and cattle, Dr. Duncan moved to Austin, Texas, and opened her own dog and cat practice. In addition to private practice, she also works extensively with local humane societies, teaches at a community college, and lends support to her husband's cow-calf operation.

It is her belief that the more informed future veterinarians become about all aspects of their chosen career, the more the veterinary profession as a whole will prosper. It is for this reason that she wrote *Careers in Veterinary Medicine*.

# Contents

# Foreword

As one of Dr. Duncan's mentors at the University of Illinois, I recognize her sincere interest in and sensitivity to her chosen profession and laud her decision to provide a realistic and well-organized guide for those interested in pursuing a career in veterinary medicine. In sharing her trials, tribulations, and philosophies as she prepared for her career, Dr. Duncan has developed a valuable resource for all young people who are interested in the field.

In meeting the demands of a rapidly expanding knowledge base and of delivery of high-quality medical care, the needs of the profession of veterinary medicine are changing dramatically. To help preveterinary students understand the relevance of these challenges to the profession, Dr. Duncan has provided an overview of the opportunities within veterinary medicine.

Preveterinary students should develop a broad scientific experience in the foundations of modern-day biological sciences and humanities to prepare themselves for the wide variety of career alternatives that are continually being identified for the holder of the Doctor of Veterinary Medicine degree.

Erwin Small, D.V.M., M.S.
Associate Dean and Professor
College of Veterinary Medicine
University of Illinois

# Veterinarian's Oath

Being admitted to the profession of veterinary medicine, I solemnly swear to use my scientific knowledge and skills for the benefit of society through the protection of animal health, the relief of animal suffering, the conservation of livestock resources, the promotion of public health, and the advancement of medical knowledge.

I will practice my profession conscientiously, with dignity, and in keeping with the principles of veterinary medical ethics.

I accept as a lifelong obligation the continual improvement of my professional knowledge and competence.

*Chapter* 1

# So You Want to Be a Veterinarian?

As a young adult, you should choose your life's work with extreme care and with full knowledge of its demands as well as its rewards. A multitude of career possibilities are open to you. Since you chose to read this book, you must be considering a future in veterinary medicine. Why? The reasons for choosing veterinary medicine as a career are almost as numerous as the people who enter the profession. Although veterinary medicine is a specialized branch of health care, it includes many tremendously diverse occupations. Few people, even those desiring to become veterinarians, are aware of all the various and sundry branches of veterinary medicine.

The upbringing and background of animal doctors varies greatly among veterinarians. Each has his own reasons for entering the profession. You, too, have unique interests and goals. Perhaps you own cherished pets and, finding enjoyment in your animals, feel that you would find satisfaction working with animals as a career. Possibly you were raised on a farm or ranch and enjoy working with livestock or horses. Maybe your goals are altruistic, and you'd like to dedicate your life to helping defenseless animals. Are you a nature lover? Some veterinarians work solely with wild animals, enabling mankind to better understand our undomesticated friends. Or are your interests more academically oriented? Perhaps you envision yourself teaching in veterinary school. Do you enjoy science, biology, and chemistry? You can find fulfillment doing research in one of the many branches of veterinary medicine.

1

At this precise moment, you are the sum total of all your previous experiences. They will determine your satisfaction with your career choice. Few professions offer as many options as veterinary medicine.

As a young person interested in veterinary medicine, try to get a good overall view of the profession. Some aspects of veterinary medicine are brand-new and offer unlimited opportunities to the veterinarian who pioneers in these areas. Other branches are "tried and true" and offer stable, satisfying careers. Some areas of the profession are actually becoming less attractive either because of oversaturation of veterinarians or because of obsolete methodology. Let's examine some of these various areas to see which have potential for growth.

First, our companion (pet) animals will provide a growing demand for more and better veterinary services. Look at current social trends. Americans are enjoying a shorter workweek, earlier retirement, and a lengthening life expectancy. As a result, an increase in the number of pets is anticipated. Better equipped, more specialized hospitals will be needed to treat these pets. Horses, after a sharp decline in number in the 1940s and 1950s, have staged a tremendous comeback as recreational animals. The horse doctor now plays a modern role in equine health care. Pet birds are increasing in number as well as in cost. Currently few veterinarians are qualified to treat these birds. More avian practitioners are needed both as specialists and as part of general small animal practices.

Medical insurance for pets is becoming popular and may have a major impact on the veterinary industry. Pet health insurance will allow more owners to afford treatment for an illness or accident that would otherwise be financially devastating for the family. Animals contract the same illnesses as people, and medical care for these illnesses costs the same for them as for people. Accidents happen all too frequently to pets. A dog that has been hit by a car may have several fractured bones. The cost for treatment may amount to several hundred or even thousands of dollars. With insurance, more pets will receive medical care instead of being put to sleep.

Psychiatrists and social workers now recognize the importance of pets to the physical and emotional well-being of the young, the aged, the lonely, and the handicapped. Caring for companion animals teaches children tenderness, responsibility, and respect for living creatures. Tests have demonstrated that simply petting an animal lowers blood pressure. The soothing purr of a cat calms upset nerves. Today's fast-paced society can use all the serenity it can find. Nursing homes, retirement centers, and mental health facilities are not only allowing small pets but encouraging such ownership. Owning a pet gives the elderly a feeling of being needed. This sense of responsibility enables some people to enjoy longer, more meaningful lives.

During the nineteenth and the first half of the twentieth century virtually all veterinary activities were associated with livestock and agriculture. Today, although the profession has become multifaceted, veterinary medicine and agriculture are still interdependent.

Maintaining adequate food supplies for human beings is the responsibility of veterinarians. Fifty percent of the food we eat is derived from animals in the form of meat and dairy products. The increasing human population will require additional food-producing animals. Much of the world has an insufficient amount of animal protein, especially low-cost animal protein. By the time the world population reaches eight billion in fifty to sixty years—double the 1975 population of four billion—the demand for food will also have doubled. In less than seventy years the human population will need an increase in food production equal to what previously took 12,000 to 14,000 years to develop. And remember, livestock are not raised only for food. They also supply much of our clothing (in the form of wool, mohair, leather, and furs). Modern food animal veterinarians should be regarded as partners in the livestock industry. Besides treatment of injuries and illnesses, current large-animal medicine involves increasing the livestock producer's profitability through preventive medicine, herd health programs, and development of an overall plan for nutrition, breeding, shelter, environment, and husbandry.

While veterinary medicine has made significant gains in controlling diseases of livestock, many more advances are required to minimize the current $3 billion annual loss to the livestock industry. Much of this loss is due to preventable diseases. Research in disease control and prevention will continue to expand. Modern

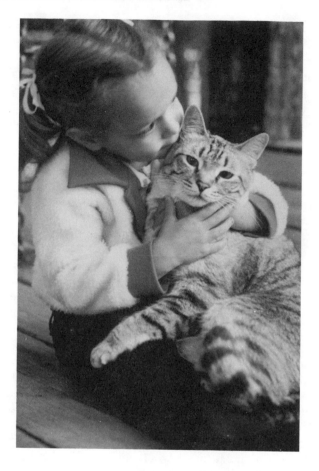

agriculture must rely on scientific and technical advancements.
An interesting development in agriculture is the possibility of
"mini" livestock. After seventeen years of experimentation, researchers at the National Autonomous University of Mexico have
successfully bred minicows. The original breed was the Indo-
Brazilian zebu, which stands almost 6 feet tall and weighs up to
2,000 pounds. The newly developed dwarf version weighs an average of 300 pounds and is 2 to 3 feet in height. These minicows produce more milk proportionate to their size than their full-sized
ancestors. The hope is that experimentation with minilivestock

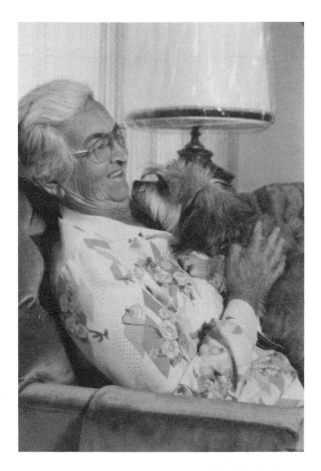

*Norden Laboratories, Inc.*
Pets are important to the physical and emotional well-being of the young and the aged.

will create low-cost animals that can be easily maintained in a small amount of space. Perhaps someday small farmyards will be stocked with miniature cattle, pigs, and fowl.

Although veterinary medicine began centuries ago as a healing art, it now reaches into many other areas. Veterinarians serve society in many ways besides doctoring pets and improving livestock production. For instance, drugs and toxic chemicals are increasing in their significance to the meat-consuming population. The public has to be protected from meat and dairy products contaminated with pesticides, hormones, antibiotics, and so on. This includes beef, pork, milk, cheese, eggs, and poultry. When new drugs or chemicals are developed for livestock, they must be stringently tested by veterinarians to insure public safety.

Also of increasing importance is the effect on animals of radiation and nuclear fallout. Research is desperately needed in this branch of veterinary medicine. Every nuclear test that is run and every nuclear plant that is built potentially affects the security of our food supply. If radiation contaminates the hay the cow eats, how safe is it to drink the milk she produces? What would happen to U.S. food supplies if a situation similar to the Soviet Union's Chernobyl accident happened in this country?

In addition, veterinarians need to formulate a nationwide plan in case of nuclear war. They will be of vital importance in the recovery phase. Initially, countless numbers of helpless animals will be wounded, burned, irradiated, and starving. Livestock deaths will immediately curtail food for humans in the form of animal protein. Reduced quantities of feed will be available to the surviving livestock because of destroyed pastures and crops. This drastic decrease in food supplies will create long-term problems even in countries not directly involved in a so-called limited nuclear war. Even after all the losses are taken into consideration, the question will remain whether the milk, eggs, and meat from the surviving animals will be safe for human consumption? Veterinarians will be called upon to supply the answers.

Biomedical research is an expanding branch of veterinary medicine. Veterinary biological research includes animal diseases that are similar to human diseases (known as animal disease models). Many animal conditions, such as genetic problems or abnormal skeletal development, closely resemble human health problems and can be used as models. For instance, veterinarians are currently using two animal viruses (the feline leukemia virus, which causes a leukemic syndrome in cats, and a virus known as SIV, which causes an immunodeficiency in monkeys) as models for the AIDS virus. Scientists have deciphered the genetic codes of these viruses. Once the detailed genetic makeup of feline leukemia and SIV are known, scientists can develop experimental vaccines, and such work should guide in development of AIDS vaccine for humans. You yourself can look forward to a longer, healthier life thanks, in part, to veterinarians.

Veterinarians will also be expected to apply their expertise to new and emerging fields such as radiation biology, genetic engineering, bioengineering, gene-splicing, embryo fusion, and cellular and molecular biology. The ultimate goal of biotechnology techniques is to produce more productive, more efficient, and more disease-resistant livestock to help alleviate the world's food shortage. Genetic research will allow scientists to take the best of a set of genetic characteristics and rearrange them to enable

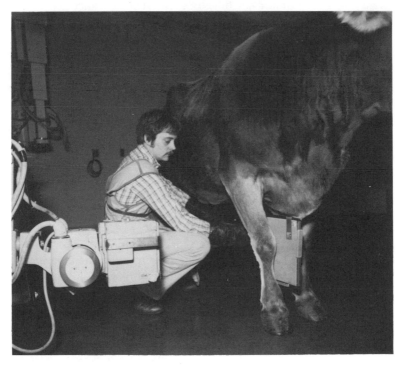

*University of Illinois College of Veterinary Medicine*
Radiology being performed on a cow.

animals to do things they normally could not do. For example, experimental pigs are currently being implanted with a reproducible human growth gene. Although these genetically altered hogs do indeed produce leaner meat, they also develop crippling arthritis as a side effect, Obviously more research is needed in this area before such pigs are incorporated into our food chain. Another example of a genetically engineered animal is a "geep," developed at the University of California–Davis when researchers fused the embryos of a goat and a sheep. Such biotechnology is in its infancy and as yet has no practical applications. However, research veterinarians have great expectations for bioengineering. Besides helping relieve world hunger, scientists are hoping such research will someday aid in our understanding of human and animal development, including abnormal development such as cancer.

Obviously the veterinary profession is an expanding one, and its future seems bright in many ways. One dark side is that an excess of veterinarians is predicted by the end of this decade. Some veterinary economists feel that the supply is going to outstrip the demand for their services. For this reason, future veterinarians must keep an open mind to the newer avenues of veterinary medicine. Overall, the outlook for veterinary medicine is still promising, and the profession offers many opportunities to the dedicated person.

If you decide to follow the path that leads to becoming an animal doctor, what lies ahead? The initial challenge will be your education. Good grades are necessary to become a veterinarian. In fact, many years of good grades are necessary. Did you realize that a veterinarian receives the same number of years of schooling as a physician? The average veterinarian completes eight years of college before he receives a diploma in veterinary medicine. That means that the young person going directly from high school into college will be (on the average) twenty-six years of age before he can actually be called a veterinarian.

By the way, the use of the pronoun *he* does not in any way suggest that this book applies only to males. It is used for simplicity's sake. In fact, in recent years the entering classes at veterinary schools have been approximately 50 percent women, and that percentage seems to be increasing.

So many years of college can be a depressing prospect to many young people. Perhaps you are one of these energetic persons who are anxious to get into "the real world" and begin pursuing the career of their dreams: lives to be saved, wounds to be healed, medical advancements to be achieved. Patience is a virtue that every animal doctor needs. Those years of school are not wasted time. They enable the aspiring veterinarian slowly and methodically to absorb the principles of the life sciences. His brain as well as his psyche becomes saturated with the tenets, theories, and precepts that govern the veterinary branch of medicine. He graduates with an aggregate knowledge of the animal kingdom. He can realistically integrate the various facets of nutrition, biochemistry, pharmacology, physiology, and genetics into a unified whole. He can view life on earth in its entirety and realize that veterinary medicine is only a minuscule portion of that whole.

My high school biology instructor told the class on the first day of school that it was his desire by the end of the semester to have each of us realize the close resemblance between ourselves and a blade of grass. Although I failed to grasp the significance of his insights in just thirty weeks of high school biology, I remembered his statement later in my academic career. Truly, when the science of life studies is appreciated to its fullest degree, the similarities, kinship, and dependency of all earth's living creatures are marvelously apparent.

The years spent in college allow time for not only the nurturing of the intellect but also the maturing of the individual. No matter how mature you may feel when you reach eighteen or twenty years old, few people at that age are capable of coping with the realities of a profession that demands immense responsibility. Should you decide to deal with the public in private practice, your clients will expect a mature doctor capable of adult communication. If you decide to enter the veterinary branch of the military or private industry, your doctor's degree will immediately place you at an upper entry level. Your subordinates will expect not only a knowledgeable veterinarian but also a fully developed person whom they can respect. This overall development of an individual takes time, and the years devoted to scholastic achievement allow for that time. Studies are designed to promote the student's professional identity, including a commitment to lifelong learning and service to clients and communities.

Those years of college are not easy. Good grades, persistence, dedication to a goal, and sacrifice must accompany each and every year. The students who are selected to enter veterinary college are the cream of the crop, so to speak. Only the top students, the ones with the best grades, graduate as veterinarians. Modern veterinary schools have been in existence only a little over a hundred years. In that century more advances have been made in veterinary medicine than during all the previous history of the profession. Obviously, there is a lot to learn while in veterinary college. The degree awarded is the Doctor of Veterinary Medicine, or D.V.M. (the exception is the University of Pennsylvania, which awards a V.M.D.)

Completion of the professional degree alone does not entitle the graduate veterinarian to practice. Each state in the U.S. sets certain standards and qualifications that the professional person must meet. Before the veterinarian can practice in a given state he must pass that state's licensing examination. Only with both a diploma and a license can a veterinarian actually begin a career.

Having devoted enormous amounts of time, money, and energy to his chosen profession, the new veterinarian is ready to tackle his first job. The majority of new graduates enter private practice. For them, an exciting career is waiting, complete with long, tiring hours. The average veterinarian in private practice (livestock, horses, or pets) devotes well over forty hours a week to his work. Many veterinarians work sixty hours a week. Those hours do not include the emergency calls during "off hours."

A veterinarian is a respected professional, looked upon as an authority in his field. His advanced training and specialized knowledge qualify him as an expert in animal health. Since he is regarded as an expert, he can expect to be compensated with a good income. A veterinarian can expect to maintain a comfortable standard of living based on his earning capabilities. But there is another side of the coin to consider.

What exactly does adequate financial compensation mean? The typical veterinarian fresh out of school in the mid-1980s earns between $15,000 and $25,000, with the average just under $24,000. Although earnings increase as the veterinarian gains additional skills and knowledge, the typical veterinarian can never expect to approach the earning capability of the M.D. Based on the accompanying table, the average 1985 earnings (before taxes) of all U.S. veterinarians with at least six years of experience was $56,000. Compare this to the average $129,200 of an experienced doctor of human medicine or the $90,600 of an experienced dentist. Yet the amount of training that goes into all three professions is not very different. A sincere devotion to both the pursuit of knowledge and the humane treatment of animals is required if the veterinarian hopes to be able to emotionally overcome the discrepancies in income. The veterinarian's unwavering concern for animals must

## COMPARISON OF SALARIES
### (1985 Average Annual Take-home Pay, Including Bonuses and Commissions)

| Occupation | Starting Salary | Salary After 6 Years |
| --- | --- | --- |
| Accountant | $23,900 | $31,700 |
| Advertising executive | $13,500 | $54,700 |
| Airline pilot | $55,000 | $110,000 |
| Chemist | $39,600 | $56,900 |
| Commercial banker | $28,550 | $54,600 |
| Computer programmer | $20,800 | $54,600 |
| Dentist | $55,000 | $90,600 |
| Electrician, unionized | $14,800 | $40,100 |
| Grade school teacher | $16,900 | $31,300 |
| Lawyer | $48,000 | $225,000 |
| Librarian | $18,000 | $31,300 |
| Life insurance agent | $15,900 | $52,600 |
| Mail carrier | $20,100 | $27,100 |
| Newspaper reporter | $19,100 | $29,800 |
| Paralegal | $16,000 | $35,000 |
| Physician | $78,900 | $129,200 |
| Professor | $26,700 | $44,600 |
| Social worker | $18,000 | $24,000 |
| Stockbroker | $35,600 | $79,600 |
| Veterinarian | $23,900 | $56,000 |

*Source*: Walterscheid, Ellen, "Which Profession Pay the Most?" *Money;* a division of Time Inc.

be present even when the work hours are inconvenient or good financial compensation is lacking.

If these challenging aspects of your chosen career have not frightened you away, perhaps you will become a top-notch veterinarian. The profession can offer positive and uplifting experiences to the person who chooses his career carefully. Without question, veterinary medicine can be tremendously rewarding and emotionally fulfilling. The joy of watching a newborn creature seek its mother for food and comfort is indescribable. The satisfaction of helping an injured animal overcome its suffering is without comparison. Discovering ways to enable God's creatures to live longer, healthier lives is truly gratifying.

The American public's vision of a veterinarian is reflected by the local practitioner who treats their pets or farm animals. This is a superficial image and an inaccurate representation of the veterinary profession. Veterinarians are involved in many activities besides doctoring animals. Veterinary medicine encompasses much more than most people realize. The primary responsibilities of the profession are twofold: to protect animal health and to protect human health. When a veterinarian receives his degree, he takes the Veterinarian's Oath. In doing so, he solemnly swears to "use his scientific knowledge and skills for the benefit of society through the protection of animal health, the relief of animal suffering, the conservation of livestock resources, the promotion of public health, and the advancement of medical knowledge." Obviously, a veterinarian who takes this oath has responsibilities that far surpass treating worms in puppies and runny noses in horses.

A career in veterinary medicine requires strong vocational motivation and dedication. It is a demanding yet rewarding profession. I hope that the following pages will make your road to becoming an animal doctor a little less rocky. As a veterinarian myself, I have tried to present my insights into the profession in an unbiased, unadorned, and straightforward fashion.

# Chapter II

# Education

Diagrammed below are the educational steps necessary to become a veterinarian. This chapter will examine each stage in more detail.

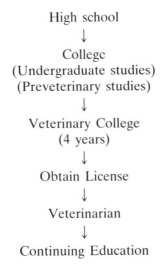

High school
↓
College
(Undergraduate studies)
(Preveterinary studies)
↓
Veterinary College
(4 years)
↓
Obtain License
↓
Veterinarian
↓
Continuing Education

*High School*

For the young person who decides early in life that he wants to pursue a career in veterinary medicine, preparation can begin in high school. Many years of college lie ahead, and good study habits must be developed. Although veterinary colleges place the greatest emphasis on the applicant's undergraduate college grades, they may also examine the grades and level of courses the student was capable of attaining in high school. Certain personal attributes can be developed while in high school that can remain with a person throughout his lifetime. The future veterinarian should develop an inquisitive mind. Learning the efficient use of time is an essential. The student needs to develop perseverance and dedication to goals.

The prospective veterinary student should take all the high school science courses available. Although the courses vary from school to school, biology, chemistry, physics, physiology, health, and zoology are recommended. Study of the sciences will not only prepare the student for college courses but also allow him to realize early in his education whether he has an aptitude for science and, therefore, medicine. If advanced or accelerated science courses are offered, the student should take them. Later in his academic career he will be competing with top students; he may as well get used to it now. The future veterinarian should especially enjoy and get good grades in biology, because essentially veterinary school is nothing more than an intensive series of specialized biology courses.

Advanced math courses, including trigonometry and calculus, will provide invaluable preparation for college-level physics and chemistry. Of course, the typical college preparatory courses such as social sciences and foreign language should be included. Among languages, Latin is an excellent choice. Although it has been considered a "dead language" and of little practical use, it is the foundation language on which medical terminology is based.

Also recommended is a typing course. The prospective veterinarian faces a minimum of six years of college, during which many papers and reports will need to be typed. Typing skill is also needed for even basic computer usage. Since computers have infiltrated practically every business and profession, including veterinary medicine, basic programming and word processing are almost essential.

Extracurricular activities should not be overlooked. Future veterinarians are encouraged to gain experience in high school through participation in 4-H, Future Farmers of America, biology clubs, and science fairs. Even students who plan to work with dogs and cats as a career would be wise to gain some experience in large animal husbandry. For one thing, veterinary schools look favorably on a well-rounded background, and for another, all veterinary school curricula include both large animals and pets. Until the 1960's the vast majority of veterinary students came from rural backgrounds. Although that is no longer true, familiarity with horse and livestock terminology and the proper safety procedures to use around these species will make the later years in veterinary school that much easier.

The high school counselor should be included in the student's plans and efforts. Counselors genuinely want to help the student and may have valuable suggestions to offer. They are experienced in helping students plan classes, choose colleges and majors, and obtain financial assistance. Counselors may have connections with the local business community and be able to help the student find an animal-related job. They can help the prospective veterinarian avoid the mistakes other students have made. They have access to career testing that can reveal a student's strengths and aptitudes. The counselor's knowledge is there to be used and is free for the asking.

*College*

Undergraduate college studies should be in direct preparation for veterinary college. Students should plan their studies to prepare them for entrance into the veterinary program.

Each veterinary college has undergraduate requirements that must be met for admission. Many veterinary schools require a minimum of sixty semester hours of preveterinary courses; some require ninety or more semester hours. Completion of these required courses usually takes two to three years of full-time study. The average student has completed four years of college before being admitted to veterinary school, and some have obtained a master's degree or a doctorate.

A list of U.S. and Canadian colleges of veterinary medicine is given in the Appendix. Information about entrance requirements can be obtained directly from them. Although the requirements vary from university to university, the following are fairly typical preveterinary courses necessary to gain entrance into veterinary school.

Biology            Botany
Microbiology       Chemistry

| | |
|---|---|
| Genetics | Organic chemistry |
| Zoology | Mathematics |
| Animal Nutrition | Physics |
| Animal Science | Social Sciences |
| Biochemistry | English (communication skills) |

The choice of college is at the student's discretion so long as it has a good academic reputation and strong science and animal science departments. In choosing a college, the student must take his own circumstances into consideration. Can his family afford a private school? Is the student responsible for financing his own education? What scholarship or financial aid is available? Is the student emotionally mature enough to live on campus away from his family?

Although every university that has a veterinary college also offers the required preveterinary courses, preference for admission is not given to graduates of that university's undergraduate school. However, attending the university where the student hopes to attend veterinary school does have certain advantages. First, being familiar with the campus means less of cultural shock for the first-year veterinary student. Second, these universities usually have substantial animal science departments, which many liberal arts colleges do not have. The student may even be able to secure part-time employment in the animal science department. The really fortunate student lands a job at the college's veterinary clinic, where he can become familiar with the faculty and the facilities. Finally, universities associated with veterinary colleges have enough students to justify a Pre-Vet Club, where ideas, information, and encouragement can be exchanged.

The student's choice of college majors is quite broad. He can major in the conventional sciences including biology, chemistry, preveterinary medicine, premedicine, predentistry, molecular biology, neurobiology, biochemistry, biomedical engineering, zoology, genetics, microbiology, or pharmacy. Alternatively he can concentrate his efforts in the school of agriculture, pursuing such majors as animal science, dairy science, poultry production, swine production, agricultural education, agricultural biochemistry, animal ecology, or fisheries and wildlife biology.

In choosing a major the student should fully realize that he has less than a fifty-fifty chance of being accepted into veterinary college. Therefore, the major he selects should lend itself to other career possibilities. In fact, veterinary schools encourage students to have an alternative career plan, to avoid developing "tunnel vision" with the only goal in sight being admission to veterinary college. During his undergraduate education he should consider alternative occupations such as teaching, livestock management, medical technology, or even human medicine.

Competition for admission to veterinary college is stiff. At each school the admissions committee is the group of school administrators who determine the prerequisites for admission and judge which students will be admitted.

The key factor the committees consider is grades, which are judged by grade point average. The grade point average is determined by adding the grades from all courses taken and dividing the total by the number of courses. For example, a B in Algebra, a B in Biology, and an A in English result in a grade point average of 3.33 (3 + 3 + 4 ÷ 3). This simplified example demonstrates the theory behind the average.

A = 4 points
B = 3 points
C = 2 points
D = 1 point

Some veterinary colleges require a minimum undergraduate grade point average of 2.5, but most have higher requirements. The typical grade point average of students currently being accepted into veterinary colleges nationwide is 3.5. In other words, the average student maintained a B+ average throughout his undergraduate studies. Students who maintained straight A's in their preveterinary courses are not uncommon.

Veterinary colleges tend to place greater emphasis on good grades in science courses than in others. Also, they may overlook a poor start in college if the student demonstrated marked improvement during the later part of his undergraduate studies. Admissions committees also prefer students who maintained a high grade point average while taking a full course schedule. The professional curriculum in veterinary school demands full-time studies of sixteen to twenty hours per semester, and preveterinary students are expected to demonstrate that they can maintain that schedule.

Another criterion used to evaluate applicants is their scores on standardized examinations such as the Graduate Record Examination (GRE), the Medical College Admissions Test (MCAT), and the Veterinary Admissions Test (VAT). These tests are offered several times yearly in many locations across the country. The test required varies from university to university. That information can be obtained directly from the university, along with information on when and where the tests are held.

Veterinary colleges look at other factors besides grades and test scores. They also use subjective criteria based on personal interviews and letters of recommendation. They try to find persons who took an active part in their community and undergraduate school, persons who demonstrate qualities of leadership, maturity, initiative, enthusiasm, poise, and the ability to get along with others.

Reading and comprehension skills are an integral part of the veterinarian's lifelong study. The practice of veterinary medicine requires competence in the spoken and written language. Candidates should be capable of expressing their thoughts effectively. For these reasons, the admissions committee evaluates applicants' communication skills.

Some universities require previous experience with a veterinarian or in a field closely related to veterinary medicine. States spend large sums of money educating veterinary students; they want to make certain that graduates remain productive members of the profession. For this reason, almost all veterinary colleges require some hands-on experience prior to admission.

Either in high school or college the candidate needs to get a part-time job on weekends or in summer vacations. This may be harder than it sounds. Such jobs are in great demand, and many students are willing to volunteer their time or work for minimum wage. Many veterinarians are glad to help students, but the students outnumber available veterinarians.

The admissions committee also looks favorably on experience involving breeding, rearing, feeding, and showing various kinds of animals, including companion animals, livestock, laboratory animals, zoo animals, or wildlife. This is where 4-H and FFA membership is helpful.

Many admissions procedures include a personal interview with applicants. This one-on-one interaction allows the committee members to evaluate the student subjectively. They can assess how well he handles himself. They see if he has a pleasing personality and appearance. They gain insights into his motivation, dedication, interests, and personal characteristics. They determine his command of the spoken language.

Veterinary schools do not discriminate on the basis of sex, religion, age, race, marital status, ethnic background, or social status. However, they do expect students to be in good health. Handicapped persons should not hesitate to apply for admission but should be honest with themselves in assessing the limitations imposed by the handicap. Admission evaluators will consider and make judgment on any handicap that would appear to affect the applicant's ability to carry out the professional activities of a veterinarian.

In 1984 approximately 43 percent of all qualified applicants were accepted into colleges of veterinary medicine. Competition is keen. In fact, many students who were rejected by veterinary schools have gone on to obtain their M.D. degree. Candidates should not be discouraged if they are not accepted with their first application. A large percentage of veterinary students gain admission only after their second or third try. Although the competition is stiff, however, it is easing slightly.

In summary, the following are the criteria that most colleges of veterinary medicine use to select students:

- Sixty to ninety undergraduate semester hours.
- Successful completion of required courses.
- High grade point average.
- Experience in the veterinary profession.
- Outstanding personal qualities and characteristics.

When a student has completed the prerequisite courses and has undergone the required testing, he can apply for admission to a college of veterinary medicine. He fills out an application, which is usually several pages in length. The deadline for return of the application is usually the fall before the year he hopes to enter veterinary school. Many colleges require that a nonrefundable fee accompany the application.

The choice of veterinary schools is limited. Only thirty-one currently are in operation in the United States and Canada. If a veterinary college is located in the applicant's home state, that is probably the only school to which he has a chance of gaining admission (unless he has very exceptional qualifications). If the student lives in a state that does not have a veterinary school, he should apply to schools with which his state has admissions agree-ments. High school or college counselors have this information. Veterinary schools must limit their students this way because the student's tuition pays only a fraction of the cost of his education. The schools rely heavily on funds from state taxes, and the state taxpayers want the funds to go toward the education of their residents.

Some schools have agreements with other states to accept a limited number of their students. Under such contractual agree-ments, the contracting state must pay the difference between what the student pays in tuition and the true cost of his education.

Many undergraduate students resent the fact that admission to veterinary school is so difficult and feel that more schools should be built. However, they need to consider the other side of the coin. Economic studies project an excess number of veterinarians within the next decade. One must remember the law of supply and demand. Why should millions of dollars be invested in establishing schools to produce veterinarians who will not be able to find jobs? More veterinary schools would place higher tax burdens on al-ready overburdened taxpayers. Some schools are actually decreas-ing the number of students they accept.

During the school years so much of the student's time, ambi-tion, and energy is spent trying to get into veterinary school that he may forget his two original goals. The first goal is *not* to become a veterinary student; it is to become a veterinarian. The second goal is to acquire a strong basic education. Admission into veterinary school may become such a priority in the student's mind that ac-ceptance into the professional college becomes the ultimate target.

## Veterinary College

Every year approximately 2,300 aspiring veterinarians are ad-mitted into professional programs nationwide. Statistically, the average first-year veterinary student is twenty-three years old, has completed four years of college, and has maintained a B+ average. Approximately 50 percent are women (or, to word it another way, about half are men).

What can these students expect during the next four years? A lot. A lot of time spent in the classroom, a lot of tests, a lot of note-taking, a lot of hours of study, a lot of money spent on books and tuition, a lot of knowledge to be crammed into their brains. The only thing veterinary students don't get a lot of is sleep.

By and large, all U.S. and Canadian veterinary schools operate on similar principles. Veterinary schools must meet certain standards set by the Council on Education of the American Veterinary Medical Association (AVMA). The colleges maintain continual liaison with each other through the Association of Deans of the American College of Veterinary Medicine. A high degree of standardization is maintained in areas such as entrance requirements, teaching methods, curricula, research facilities, and libraries. Because of this, all veterinary schools provide their graduates with an adequate education. Whereas one school may have brand-new buildings and facilities and another may have a reputation for an exceptional equine department, veterinary students need not worry whether their particular school is giving them a top-notch education.

At all veterinary colleges the first two years are devoted largely to classroom studies. Students find themselves in the classroom almost eight hours a day plus spending many evenings in the anatomy or histology laboratory. They devote many hours daily to homework and after-school studies. Textbooks, note-taking, homework, and written tests continue just as they did in college. Basic principles of animal biology are reviewed and expanded upon.

The student first learns to identify the healthy animal. What does the healthy Thoroughbred look like? The healthy Great Dane? The healthy billy goat? What does healthy skin look like? Healthy feathers? Healthy hooves? How about healthy eyes? Healthy brain? Healthy blood? What does normal manure from a healthy animal look like? One must be able to identify "normal" in order to recognize "abnormal." The study of the abnormal animal is termed pathology and includes the identification of disease processes, their causes, symptoms, progression, effects, and treatment. In order to recognize the normal and the abnormal, the healthy and the unhealthy, the following subjects must be mastered during the first half of veterinary school:

Anatomy—study of the body structure of animals

Physiology—study of the functions and vital life processes of animals

Embryology—study of the formation and development of animals before they are born (developmental anatomy)

Histology—microscopic study of tissues and cells (microscopic anatomy)

Animal science—general study of various animals, their nutrition, reproduction, environmental needs, economic value

Microbiology and virology—study of bacteria, fungi, and viruses and the diseases they cause

Genetics—study of inheritable characteristics

Pharmacology—study of drugs

Epidemiology—study of the interrelationships between the animal, its environment, and disease-producing organisms or substances

Parasitology—study of parasites such as worms, fleas, and ticks

Immunology—study of protection against disease, such as vaccination

Radiology—study of X rays and their uses

Toxicology—study of poisonous substances and plants

Theriogenology—study of animal reproduction

Anesthesiology—study of tranquilizers and drugs used to put an animal to sleep for surgery

Surgical principles—basic theories governing surgery

The course that seems to spark the most interest in visitors to the veterinary school is anatomy, which is usually taken in the freshman year. Students are divided into groups of three, four, or five. At the beginning of the semester they dissect a dog or a cat or both. Later in the year they dissect a horse and a cow. Dissection of even a small animal may take a couple of months. Every nerve, every muscle, every blood vessel must be isolated and identified, which can be quite an undertaking in a 900-pound cow! Preservative keeps the tissues relatively soft and pliable. The anatomy lab can present quite a grotesque picture to anyone who is not a veterinary student. A dog cadaver lies on each table and preserved horses and cattle hang from hoists around the room.

In addition to macroscopic anatomy, students spend many hours on microscopic anatomy. Under a microscope each body tissue has a different appearance from all other tissues. A spleen looks vastly different from a liver. A kidney does not even resemble an ovary. Students must be able to identify every body part microscopically and know whether it is in a healthy or a diseased state.

Freshman and sophomore students also spend a lot of time looking through microscopes at disease-producing organisms. The air we breathe, the food we eat, the things we touch are full of microorganisms, some of which are pathogenic, that is, capable of producing disease. The majority are harmless. Veterinarians have to be able to microscopically identify all disease-producing organisms, including ectoparasites (fleas, lice, mange mites...),

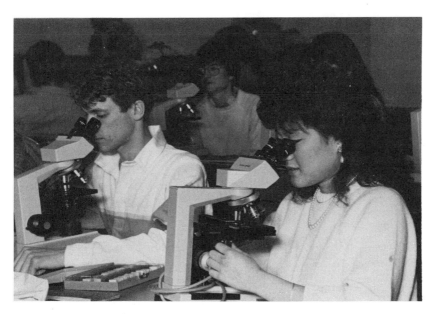

*University of Illinois College of Veterinary Medicine*
Students look at slides through microscopes.

endoparasites (roundworms, heartworms, flukes...), bacteria (*Salmonella, E. coli, Pseudomonas*...), fungi (*Microsporum canis, Blastocyces dermatitidis, Coccidioides immitus*...), and protozoa (*Eimeria bovis, Toxoplasma gondii, Giardia lamblia*...).

All students must learn about horses, dogs, cats, birds, cows, pigs, sheep, and goats, whether they have an interest in that species or not. The woman from New York must learn to handle and treat cattle just as the rancher's son from Oklahoma must deal with parakeets. In the later part of the curriculum a limited number of elective courses are available in which the student may follow his particular interests.

Veterinary students are on a nine-month schedule in the freshmen and sophomore years, allowing two summers with no classes. Wise students take advantage of this time off to gain additional veterinary experience and try to apply some of their book learning. These prospective veterinarians work for minimum wage at best. Some veterinarians offer room and board to students in lieu of wages.

Upon successful completion of the first two years the student receives a Bachelor of Veterinary Medicine degree and the privilege of pursuing knowledge of a more clinical nature. Although the student has not escaped from the classroom entirely, he does gain more practical experience in surgery and clinical medicine in the college's veterinary hospital during the remaining two years. He is taught to apply the knowledge he acquired as a freshman and sophomore.

Students are assigned cases for which they are responsible just as if they were working in a private clinic. The aspiring veterinarian gets his first taste of being on call for emergencies or staying up all night with a sick animal. Students "rotate" through the various clinics at the college's hospital. They may work with horses for six weeks, then treat dogs and cats, then perfect their radiology skills. They spend a period of time making farm calls. They master basic surgery such as spays and castrations and acquire the fundamental skills to perform more complex surgery such as bone plating and cataract removal. Several weeks may be spent in the necropsy block learning to dissect dead animals and identify the cause of their illness or death. The students are divided into groups for these rotations through the clinics. These groups, under the professors' supervision, are responsible for keeping the hospital running smoothly every day of the year.

In the equine clinic of the veterinary school, each student is assigned the care of several hospitalized horses. He must diagnose their illness, devise a treatment plan, medicate, monitor their response, and exercise and groom them. Horses also come into the clinic on an outpatient basis. Outpatient visits can include pregnancy palpations, radiographing an injured leg, or diagnosing a skin disease. At the end of a day students discuss their cases with the other students on the equine rotation so that all may benefit and gain knowledge.

Students must learn how to handle a horse to avoid injury (to themselves *and* the horse). It's a rare horse that will allow a stranger to enter a stall and put a thermometer in its rectum. Proper placement and fitting of tack (saddles, bridles, bits) is practiced. Principles of restraint (twitches, stanchions, tranquilizers) are mastered. Students handle all types of horses, including brood mares, stallions, ponies, draft horses, racehorses, and pleasure horses.

Surgical techniques for horses are similar, in theory, to all surgical principles (veterinary or human) but are unique in practice because of the sheer bulk of the animal. Anesthetizing and laying a horse on a surgical table is no small task. Horses also differ from most other animals in temperament, in their high susceptibility to tetanus and other infections, and in their tendency to leg injuries, breeding problems, and digestive disorders.

The food animal ward is also located in the large animal clinic but is handled on a different rotation. The student's experience there varies somewhat depending on the region of the country. Veterinary students at the University of Wisconsin treat more dairy cows whereas other schools see more beef cattle, or sheep, or pigs, or whatever is the predominant animal of economic value in their area. These animals are hopitalized in individual stalls, and the cases are assigned to individual students. As with horses, some livestock are treated on an outpatient basis.

.Proper restraint is just as essential for livestock as it is for horses. Learning to manipulate large animal paraphernalia (gates, squeeze shoots, Iowa hog holders, electric prods, nose tongs) is the first step in food animal medicine. The techniques used in the physical examination of a bull are quite different from those used for a Persian cat. Many student toes get bruised from being stepped on in the food animal ward. Students must always remember to urinate before they treat a large animal. Sound funny? A properly placed kick to the abdomen by a Hereford will easily empty a full bladder.

The urban veterinary student is faced with a wide variety of specialized equipment made for livestock. Dehorners, Burdizzo emasculators, elastrators, ear notchers, balling guns, and hoof nippers are all found in the large animal clinic. The student must familiarize himself with the "tools of the trade." Many students get to milk a cow for the first time in their lives. Remember, a milk cow in full production has to milked twice a day, every day. Often this is the student's job.

Surgery on ruminants (sheep, goats, cattle) is different from that on horses, which is often done with the horse lying down. In ruminants, much of the abdominal surgery is performed with the animal in a standing position using only a local anesthetic.

During the farm call, or ambulatory, portion of a veterinary student's education, local farmers notify the veterinary school of their animals' needs, and the students travel to the farms. The predominant species varies with the region of the country (beef cows at Texas A & M, hogs at Iowa State University). In addition to treating farm animals, the veterinary school and its students are responsible for keeping the university's herds, packs, and flocks healthy. The ambulatory block tends to provide the experience most closely resembling an actual large animal practice. The veterinary student must brave all kinds of weather and learn to restrain and treat animals with less than optimal facilities.

For many years equine and food animal medicine comprised the bulk of a veterinarian's education. Today veterinary students spend an equal amount of time, if not more, in the small animal clinic. While on the small animal rotation, students doctor cats, dogs, birds, and many small exotic animals such as snakes and monkeys. Large exotic animals (such as a zebra from a local zoo) would be treated in the large animal clinic.

Besides sharpening their skills in diagnosis and treatment, students in the small animal clinic also practice their client communication skills. In the outpatient section, local residents bring in their pets for vaccinations, minor injuries, and illnesses. The student clinician must "work up the case," that is, talk to the client, understand the history of the sickness, list possible diagnoses, request the appropriate laboratory tests, discuss costs, and formulate a treatment regimen. This requires a lot of interaction with the owner. Building self-confidence in client communication is a slow process.

The first few times the student deals individually with an owner in an exam room are almost as frightening as the first time he makes an incision in a live animal. While on the small animal surgery rotation, students learn to perform common surgeries. Although the speed and skill with which they operate will improve with time, all employers expect the new graduate to be able to competently (though perhaps slowly) perform spays, castrations, and cat declaws. While in school, students act primarily as assistants for the more complicated operations such as orthopedic repairs, limb amputations, and spinal cord decompression. The professors do the bulk of the skilled surgery. However, open eyes and an open mind allow the future veterinarian to accumulate the practical knowledge necessary for later clinical application.

All animals regardless of species will require some overnight and emergency care. The veterinary student is on call for emergencies while on equine, food animal, ambulatory, and small animal rotations. If a horse colics (has severe abdominal pain), the student may have to come into the clinic to help perform surgery. A dog in shock from being hit by a car needs attention NOW, not in the morning. In the Intensive Care Unit of the veterinary clinic, students monitor the acutely ill patients who are in critical condition. The ICU demands constant attention. Students must skip classes, stay awake all night, miss the New Year's Eve party, or make whatever sacrifices are necessary to monitor and treat the animals.

Anesthetic techniques are mastered through practical hands-on experience. While fellow students are trying out their scalpels, student anesthesiologists keep the patients asleep. Anesthesia includes general anesthesia (totally asleep and without feeling), sedation (sleepy with pain perception still present), and local anesthesia (deadening a certain portion of the body while the animal is totally awake).

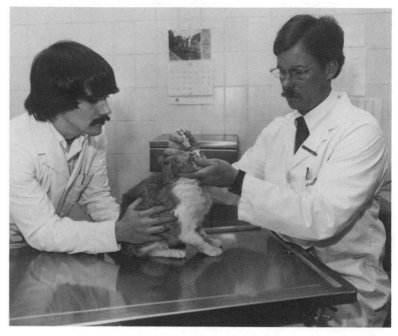

*University of Illinois College of Veterinary Medicine*
A student restrains a cat while the veterinarian applies eye drops.

Different anesthetic protocols are required for different situations. For example, the drug used on a six-month-old puppy being spayed is different from a brood bitch having a Caesarean section. The anesthetic used for a horse castration is different from that for a horse requiring minor surgery on a knee. The gases used for general anesthesia can cause miscarriage in pregnant women—an important fact that both female veterinary students and graduates need to remember.

During radiology rounds, the students practice taking radiographs on all types of animals. The principles are the same regardless of the species; the techniques vary. Horses receive the most radiographs of the large animals. Their legs are injury-prone, and a horse without good legs is undesirable even as a pet. The bulk of the student's X-ray experience is with small animals. The students practice techniques, positioning the animals, developing radiographs, interpreting the films, and performing specialized procedures such as GI series and cancer radiation. They must learn and exercise proper safety techniques. Radiation can be dangerous. This is another rotation that a pregnant student would want to avoid.

Necropsy (autopsy on animals) is a necessary yet somber portion of the veterinarian's education. Not all dead animals need to be necropsied. Sometimes, however, it is imperative that the cause of death be determined. If several laying hens die at an egg farm, the disease must be identified and stopped before the entire flock is destroyed. Sometimes thorough examination of the dead animals and use of laboratory tests is the only way a diagnosis can be obtained. Like human doctors, veterinarians are facing an increasing number of liability lawsuits. Some clients accuse their veterinarian of negligence and malpractice. Necropsies may be necessary to decide the outcome of such cases.

Precise regimens and procedures are essential to perform a necropsy so that nothing is overlooked. Organs must be handled gently so that the laboratory can then run the necessary tests on those tissues. That may be harder than it sounds considering that large, heavy saws are needed to cut open a cow's skull. If necropsy isn't the student's favorite rotation, at least there are no emergency calls and ICU duty! Besides necropsy, the students learn and practice other diagnostic laboratory services, such as clinical serology, pathology, histopathology, toxicology, bacteriology, virology, and parasitology. Any combination of these tests may be needed to determine the cause of a disease.

Unlike human medical education, no internship is presently required of veterinarians. However, most schools set aside a period of time (usually six weeks) in the senior year for gaining practical experience outside the university. These blocks of time are known as externships or preceptorships. Actual internship positions, although not required, are available after graduation with universities and large veterinary hospitals.

Some thought must be given to the costs of veterinary college. The average annual tuition in 1987 was slightly over $4,000, with a range of $1,500 to over $10,000, depending on the university. By the time this book is published and read, costs will undoubtedly have gone up. Veterinary textbooks are more expensive than those used in undergraduate studies, and fees and supplies add several hundred dollars every semester (not to mention the cost of football games, social events, and coffee for those late-night study sessions!) Some veterinary colleges require that students supply their own lab coats, surgical gloves and instruments, microscopes, hoof picks, lead ropes, and many other items.

Veterinary schools have counselors who are familiar with the financial aid programs, student loans, and scholarships. Many students borrow money to complete their education. Most veterinarians (over 80 percent) graduate from school in debt. In the mid-1980's the average veterinary school graduate completed his schooling with an educational debt close to $25,000. The veterinary professional program is rigorous and time-consuming. While some students manage to work part time and maintain good grades, most should not count on full-time employment for income for living expenses.

Veterinary school isn't all work and no play. The Student Chapter of the American Veterinary Medical Association (SCAVMA) has a branch on each veterinary campus. This organization helps provide unity among the veterinary colleges in the United States and Canada. It also assists the student in the transition between the academic and the professional worlds. Another organization is the spouses' auxiliary to SCAVMA, which is made up of wives and husbands of veterinary students and provides them with meaningful access to their spouse's veterinary career. The SCAVMA and the auxiliary plan several social events throughout the year to promote student camaraderie and to ease the tensions of study. Also on all campuses are student fraternities and special interest groups such as Christian veterinary students, students desiring to excel in bovine (cattle) medicine, students who enjoy jogging, etc. The professional curriculum does not allow time for competitive interscholastic athletics.

Finally, 5,000 classroom hours later, the student is awarded the degree of Doctor of Veterinary Medicine (D.V.M.) or, from the University of Pennsylvania, Veterinariae Medicinae Doctoris (V.M.D.) The student must now get used to being called "Doctor." He is no longer a student, but a professional. A major goal in his life has been reached. After years of hard work and sacrifice, his perseverance has finally paid off. His career as a veterinarian is about to begin.

## Licensing and Continuing Education

Each state requires that the graduate veterinarian pass a test to obtain a license to practice in that state. The purpose of the licensing examination is to insure that a certain level of quality is maintained by professionals in that state. The examination must be passed before the veterinarian can actually work as an animal doctor. Each state gives the examination at least once a year. Some states have reciprocal agreements with other states to honor their licenses. The veterinarian must pay an annual fee to keep his license. The license can be revoked if the practitioner is found guilty of incompetent or unethical behavior.

Even after the diploma and the license have been obtained, professional education must always be a part of a veterinarian's life. A veterinarian cannot attend college for eight years and then feel competent to practice the rest of his life; the profession is advancing at too rapid a rate. A conscientious veterinarian continues to expand his skills.

Many of the job options other than private practice require advanced, post-D.V.M. studies. Formal postgraduate education is available through universities. A veterinarian can earn an M.A. or a Ph.D. in areas as diverse as epidemiology or business or marine biology and use the degree in combination with the D.V.M. for teaching or research purposes.

Other veterinarians opt to complete an internship. These doctors prefer that their advanced education be strictly in clinical veterinary medicine. Besides being available at all veterinary colleges, internships are also available at several large private hospitals. The Animal Medical Center in New York and the Angell Memorial Hospital in Boston are examples of such hospitals. Internships are designed for the student who wants to pursue specific advanced studies in clinical veterinary medicine. They are in one select area, such as small animal medicine, equine medicine, or food animal medicine. Internships are limited in number and are generally open only to students who graduate from veterinary school with very good grades. Internships provide an excellent opportunity for new graduates who want to excel in their field, gain practical experience under the guidance of a specialist, and gain self-confidence. Although the intern receives a salary, it is frequently low (typically $15,000 to $16,000).

Residencies are available after internships. These involve two or three years of intensive specialized training in a limited area (e.g., ophthalmology, small animal surgery, neurology). A resident's salary is higher than that of an intern.

The American Veterinary Medical Association recognizes certain specialties in which veterinarians can become board-certified. For example, someone who is board-certified in zoological medicine is considered an expert in that field, having achieved that status through advanced education, self-study, years of experience, and passing an examination. Specialty boards currently include toxicology, laboratory animal medicine, theriogenology, anesthesiology, internal medicine, microbiology, ophthalmology, pathology, preventive medicine, radiology, veterinary practice, zoological medicine, education, dermatology, and surgery.

Most veterinarians do not include formal studies in their post-D.V.M. education. For the average practitioner, continuing education is less structured. The AVMA and the Auxiliary to the AVMA are organizations in which the veterinarian and his spouse can remain active throughout their lives. The AVMA has 44,000 members. Individual states also have Veterinary Medical Associations. Specialty organizations such as the American Animal Hospital Association, the American Association of Equine Practitioners, and the American Association of Bovine Practitioners help the veterinarian keep up-to-date with his branch of medicine. The veterinarian can also keep current with new developments through numerous professional journals.

Frequent meetings, seminars, conferences, and conventions are held at the local, national, and international levels. A scan of scheduled meetings could reveal events as diverse as meetings for the Society for Industrial Microbiology, Veterinary Cancer Society, American Embryo Transfer Association, International Conference on Veterinary Acupuncture, and International Mastitis Symposium. Essentially, a veterinarian needs to remain a student his entire professional life. The Veterinarian's Oath requires a "life-long obligation [to] the continual improvement of professional knowledge and competence." The veterinarian who doesn't continue his education stagnates.

# Chapter III

# Private Practice

Approximately three quarters of U.S. veterinarians are engaged in private practice. The private practice veterinarian can work with small animals, large animals, or both.

While still in veterinary school the student generally decides where his interests lie. Regardless of whether it is pets or farm animals, the graduate generally takes a job with an experienced veterinarian to perfect his newly acquired skills. This practical experience is essential for the young veterinarian, since his self-confidence is often low when he leaves college. Fully as much knowledge and know-how is acquired in that first year out of college as is obtained during any year of schooling. "Book learning" is only the basis; practical experience is then built upon that foundation. The importance of being associated with a high-quality veterinary practice in the first few years out of school cannot be overstressed. If can affect the veterinarian's attitude toward his profession for the rest of his career.

How does the new graduate find out about job opportunities? Most veterinary colleges maintain a file of positions that are open in private practices and with other schools and private companies. The schools rely on the private practitioners, schools, and companies to supply this information. Teachers and professors typically have wide connections with practitioners throughout the state and may recommend certain students for job openings. Some students go back to the practice where they worked while in undergraduate college or during their externship. Also, most veterinary journals have classified sections listing job opportunities and practices for sale. The AVMA publishes a list of employers and openings as well as of veterinarians seeking employment. Once the new graduate gets his first veterinary position, other job opportunities can emerge "through the grapevine" via drug salesmen, conventions, and local associations.

A typical starting salary for a new graduate is $20,000 to $25,000. As a rule veterinarians on the East Coast receive higher salaries than those who practice in the South. Veterinarians in major metropolitan areas also tend to receive higher salaries than rural practitioners. Many employers provide fringe benefits that may include employer-paid continuing education, medical insurance, liability insurance, profit-sharing and pension plans, and paid vacations.

The new graduate has plenty of time to acquire experience since the majority of veterinary positions in private practice include workweeks well over forty hours. A veterinarian's day does not end at 5:00 p.m. In fact, the nationwide trend is for veterinary clinics to be open evening hours and weekends. The majority of veterinarians also answer emergency calls nights, weekends, and holidays. The advantage of being near a metropolitan area is having access to a veterinary emergency clinic that can handle clients' emergencies when the veterinarian is unable or unwilling to be present.

Some veterinarians share responsibilities by forming group practices in which two or more doctors share the facilities and the caseload. These clinics can be owned by one veterinarian with the others working for him, or all the veterinarians can be partners in the enterprise. Not all aspects of group practice are advantageous. As in any interpersonal relationship, personality conflicts, misunderstandings, and legal problems can add tension to the clinic environment.

The majority of private practice veterinarians at some point in their career want to own their own business. They become disenchanted working for someone else and want to do things their way. They feel that the only way to make a really good income is to be on their own. The truth is that the early years of owning a veterinary clinic can be financially draining. When a veterinarian becomes self-employed he must be prepared to support himself in some way other than his veterinary practice. He should have enough money saved to meet his living expenses for two years. Lucky veterinarians have a supportive spouse who is willing to help financially during the first lean years. Generally, a clinic loses money the first six to eight months that it is open. The next one to three years are usually break-even at best.

Building a clientele is a slow, laborious process. Equipping and stocking a clinic is expensive, and most veterinarians borrow money for their initial capital. A debt of $40,000 to $100,000 is a heavy burden to carry (and a $100,000 clinic is a small clinic!). Often the neophyte veterinarian/businessman is frustrated because his receptionist earns more than he does! Some veterinarians can't afford to hire a receptionist at all and must operate a completely one-man business: veterinarian, receptionist, business manager, technician, bookkeeper, and kennel person.

Generally, a veterinary hospital is established for two to three years before it moves beyond the break-even stage to profitability. Of course, the time varies with such factors as the need for the doctor's services in a community, the location, his personal characteristics, his management expertise, and the extent of his investment and overhead. Purchasing an established clinic takes some of the sting out of those first few years of ownership. For the ambitious person who desires to have his own pet hospital, the potential rewards and responsibilities are greater than for the salaried employee.

A veterinarian who goes into business for himself must combine his medical skills with those of a businessman or entrepreneur. He must be self-motivated, be able to handle employees, make sure income is greater than expenditures, deal with dissatisfied (and sometimes irrational) clients, learn about taxes and the Internal Revenue Service, and essentially assume responsibility for every facet of the business. On the other hand, the owner-veterinarian has more control over his business environment. He can hire whomever he likes, set his own working hours, stock his clinic with equipment according to his preferences, and develop the type of practice he prefers. Being a small-business owner can be demanding, time-consuming, and emotionally draining (regardless of the type of business). It can also be gratifying, fulfilling, and financially rewarding.

*Small Animal Practitioner*

The most common image the American public has of a veterinarian is the "dog and cat doctor." In fact, approximately 40 percent of the 30,000 private practice veterinarians in the United States are engaged in small animal practice. Also known as a small animal veterinarian or small animal practitioner, he may not limit his practice just to the fifty-five million dogs and the fifty-two million cats in the United States. He may also treat pet birds, guinea pigs, rabbits, hamsters, monkeys, snakes, and turtles. Or he may limit his practice to cats (feline medicine) or dogs (canine medicine).

Small animal medicine is very demanding in the knowledge, expertise, and skills it requires. The specialty is advancing rapidly. Procedures that were considered new and innovative in human medicine twenty years ago are commonplace in veterinary medicine today. The dog and cat doctor does not just give vaccinations and treat minor problems. He has to be up-to-date on all phases of pet health.

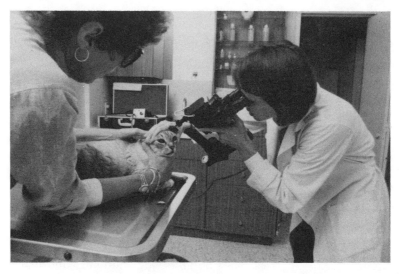

*Norden Laboratories, Inc.*
A veterinarian performs a high-tech diagnostic technique on a pet cat.

The small animal practitioner is not merely the equivalent of a general practitioner. He is also a pharmacist, surgeon, dentist, ophthalmologist, nutritionist, obstetrician, radiologist, dermatologist, laboratory technician, psychologist, anesthesiologist, and internal medicine specialist (not to mention occasional kennel person and groomer.) In exchange for these services, small animal veterinarians receive average before-tax earnings of approximately $40,000.

Just as people go to a doctor's office or a hospital for treatment, so too should animals go to a fully equipped veterinary facility to receive the best treatment possible. Only a few veterinarians still make house calls. The small animal clinic is generally one of the best-equipped veterinary facilities. Besides everyday equipment such as stethoscope and microscope, numerous specialized and expensive pieces of equipment are utilized. Ophthalmoscopes are important for examining pets' eyes. Radiograph machines are practically essential. Equipment to perform blood analysis is indispensable for establishing a diagnosis. Urinalysis can be mandatory in some cases. Electrocardiographs to evaluate the heart are not uncommon. Surgical instruments are naturally a part of a clinic. A huge, up-to-date drug inventory is required.

It is the opinion of many small animal veterinarians that the one-, two-, or three-person practice will be obsolete within the next few decades. These practices will be replaced by hospitals designed with concepts similar to human hospitals. The cost of equipping, staffing, operating, and paying loan interest on a small animal practice is staggering. Operating a veterinary hospital with three or fewer practitioners is not cost-effective. More and more veterinarians are realizing that their salaries will remain low unless they band together and share equipment and facilities.

If thirty or fifty veterinarians were to cooperate in a central hospital, they could have access to a decent laboratory, adequate X-ray equipment, a well-equipped surgical suite, an emergency service for nights and weekends, and all the other features of a hospital. Board-certified radiologists, surgeons, pathologists, and so on could be on the staff to offer consultation services to the general practitioners. As matters now stand, those thirty to fifty veterinarians are probably practicing in twenty to twenty-five individual clinics, none of which are adequately equipped. To put it bluntly, the patients are not receiving the best possible care, and because of high overhead the veterinarians are not receiving salaries commensurate with their professional expertise.

Each of those twenty to twenty-five clinics has an radiograph machine that is used perhaps thirty minutes per day. A more logical approach would be for all those doctors to share one radiograph machine, which could be an expensive, deluxe model, capable of better performance. Technicians experienced in radiology would be capable of properly positioning the animal and using correct radiology techniques. The same is true of the surgical room. Why build and equip a room that is used one or two hours out of every twenty-four? Why not share, as human medical doctors do? Staff veterinarians could then enjoy the advantage of having trained support personnel to assist in surgery.

Large centralized veterinary hospitals would benefit hospital owners, staff veterinarians, and patients. There would be better care, less duplication of facilities, better utilization of equipment, and greater financial return on investment. The future of the small animal clinic lies in central hospitals.

Although most pet doctors prefer to operate out of a clinic or hospital, a demand exists in some areas for the veterinarian to make house calls. Particularly in high-density urban locations or in areas with a large number of elderly or handicapped clients, a house call practice can be quite successful. Also, in modern society where both spouses work full time, many couples are willing to pay for the convenience of home service. Such a practice is known as a mobile clinic. It can be as simple as a car with a doctor's black bag or as complex as a specially designed, self-contained van complete with running water, drugs, instruments, equipment, examining table, and cages. Although some veterinarians perform routine surgery in their mobile clinic, most have a working relationship with a conventional veterinary hospital that allows them to perform operations in its surgical suite.

Let's look at a typical day in the small animal clinic. By the way, although the terms "veterinary clinic" and "veterinary hospital" are often used interchangeably, there is actually a difference. The term "clinic" can be used for any veterinary facility. A veterinary "hospital," on the other hand, must have facilities to hospitalize patients for longer than just a day. Outpatient visits usually com-

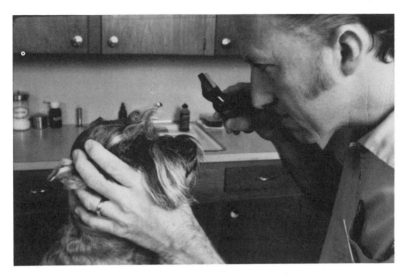

Norden Laboratories, Inc.
An eye infection is a common complaint treated by a small animal veterinarian.

prise the bulk of the work. "Outpatients" are animals brought to the clinic, treated by a veterinarian, and then taken home. New puppy examination, vaccination, flea infestation, ear infection, sore throat, worms, and minor wounds are just a few of the reasons an owner brings a pet to the doctor.

The term "inpatient" refers to all animals that stay at the hospital for longer than a day. Inpatients include animals that are hospitalized for surgery or illness. The most common surgery includes spaying (ovariohysterectomy) in female cats and dogs, neutering (castration) in male cats and dogs, and declawing of cats. Other surgical procedures are tooth extraction, orthopedics (bone repair), tumor removal, ear cropping (in breeds such as Dobermans, Great Danes, and schnauzers), removing bladder stones, retrieving foreign objects from the digestive tract, and suturing lacerations.

For commonly encountered illnesses, such as abscesses resulting from fights, urinary infections, intestinal viruses, birthing problems, and parasites, the diagnosis is relatively easy and the treatment can be carried out according to a precise regimen. However, hardly a day goes by without a case being presented to a veterinarian that causes him to scratch his head and wonder what is the cause of the illness. Even after a battery of diagnostic tests, the cause may not be determined. Or if a diagnosis is made and treatment initiated, the patient may not respond as expected. These cases remind us that medicine is an art as well as a science. Living creatures are not mechanical objects that always react in a predetermined fashion. A procedure that worked well 999 times may have undesirable results on the thousandth try. One must also consider that some diseases are untreatable and fatal.

Another circumstance occurs when an illness is expensive to treat beyond the owner's financial ability or willingness to pay for it. Some owners refuse even to have a diagnostic workup performed. It is the owner's option to have the animal destroyed even if the disease is curable. Since most veterinarians enter the profession because of their affection for animals, euthanasia (from the Greek language meaning "easy death") is a frustrating yet frequent procedure they are obligated to perform.

*Large Animal Practitioner*

Large animal practitioners are veterinarians who treat any or all of the following: horses, cattle, pigs, domestic fowl, sheep, and goats. Approximately 13 percent of the veterinarians engaged in private practice are exclusively large animal practitioners. Their patients can range from a day-old calf born to a docile milk cow to a herd of rampant beef cattle raised on a 20,000-acre ranch who have never seen a human being before. The clientele can be as diverse as a sixteen-year-old girl who owns a single pony and a farmer who feeds 1,000 hogs a year and treats them as a business. Large animal medicine can provide an exhilarating variety of animals, people, and situations. "Never a dull moment" is the byword of this practitioner.

While the sundry array of animals presented to a "country vet" can be challenging, such diversification puts an extra demand on him. He must be knowledgeable about many different species, and he must continually learn new techniques and treatments for all those animals. That is why many large animal veterinarians choose to specialize in one area: racehorses, pleasure horses, dairy cows, beef cattle, pigs, goats, and so on. Then he can be certain of doing a top-notch job. To know everything about every animal is a hopeless task; however, in many rural areas the general practitioner is expected to do exactly that.

A farm veterinarian must be a surgeon, pharmacist, nutritionist, geneticist, obstetrician, dentist, radiologist. Occasionally he is even required to function as a cowboy. He must be able to rope, tie, or otherwise restrain animals. A surprising number of ranchers have neither the workers nor the facilities to handle their livestock.

Although the small animal practitioner and the large animal practitioner have a lot in common, marked differences do exist. The large animal veterinarian averages a longer workweek than a small animal doctor, beginning his days early and working late. For instance, pigs cannot be handled during hot weather since they may suffer heat stroke. If a large number of pigs are to be vaccinated, the veterinarian must leave his office before daybreak so that he can start work as soon as the sun rises. Another example is the client who works in town but lives on a couple of acres in the country. By the time he gets home and realizes that his horse is sick it is 6:00 or 7:00 p.m. before he calls the veterinarian—who in turn does not get home until after 9:00 p.m. at the earliest.

Unlike the small animal practitioner, the large animal veterinarian cannot enjoy the comfort of a climate-controlled clinic all day. Much of his time is spent in pastures or barns regardless of the weather. Driving rainstorms, 100 degree temperatures, midnight snowstorms, and subfreezing weather require the veterinarian to be a hardy individual. Although the trend lately has been to encourage owners to haul their animals to the clinic for treatment, the "country vet" still spends a considerable number of hours driving from farm to farm. Some days he spends more hours in his car or truck than he does treating animals. In certain parts of the western United States, the veterinarian's automobile has been replaced by an airplane as he makes his calls at thousand-acre ranches.

Many large animal practitioners are trying to decrease the number of farm calls they make. Spending hours on the road is an inefficient use of a doctor's time. At a well-equipped veterinary

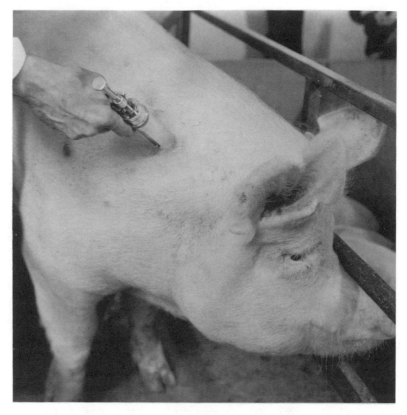

*Norden Laboratories, Inc.*
The large animal practitioner must leave his office to treat a hog at the farm.

clinic, the doctor can do a better job of diagnosis and treatment, and the clinic has better facilities for restraining the animal. Proper stanchions and squeeze shoots and a trained staff result in fewer injuries to animals and humans.

Seldom does the large animal veterinarian have use of emergency facilities; he usually handles his own after-hours calls. Horses in particular seem to have more than their share of "after dinner" problems. A multiveterinarian practice can greatly relieve the doctor of the responsibility of being on call twenty-four hours a day.

Financially, the veterinarian who deals exclusively with livestock and horses can expect an average salary of $35,000 to $45,000. The average income for strictly equine veterinarians is generally a little higher than that of veterinarians who work with livestock.

One advantage that the large animal practitioner has is the ability to open a clinic with comparatively low overhead expenses. All that is required at the beginning is a car, instruments, a mobile telephone, and portable radiograph and lab equipment. He can function out of his home or rent a small office. Over time, he can enlarge his clinic and expand his services to suit his tastes.

The workday of a large animal practitioner varies according to the species under his care. Each individual species offers a wide range of opportunities and challenges. Equine medicine, for example, is tremendously diverse: doctoring backyard pleasure horses, being a veterinarian on a large breeding farm, or dealing with racehorses. The "horse hospital" can be a barn, pasture, backyard, racetrack, or (most convenient of all) a veterinary clinic. Horse stanchions and tranquilizers can provide valuable protection from a jittery horse. Horse doctors are frequently called on to do castration (gelding), to treat injured legs, skin lacerations, and colic, and to do pregnancy testing, dental work, worming, and vaccination. Many owners carry insurance on expensive horses in case of injury or death; veterinarians are needed to examine the animal for any preexisting ailment. Racetrack veterinarians are specialists and are well compensated for their expertise. They not only treat leg injuries, insure soundness, and screen for illegal drugs but also work with the trainer to develop and fine-tune an optimum program in preparing that animal to be a winner.

Bovine (cattle) medicine commonly includes calving problems, mastitis (inflammation of the milk glands), pneumonia, digestive disorders, parasites, pregnancy testing, and foot infections. However, many differences exist within the field of bovine health care. A veterinarian in Lancaster County, Pennsylvania, works almost exclusively with dairy cattle. These cows are used to being handled by people. Many, although certainly not all, are relatively docile and easy to examine and treat. Dairy cows can usually be treated in their stanchions, whereas beef cattle can be worked in a chute

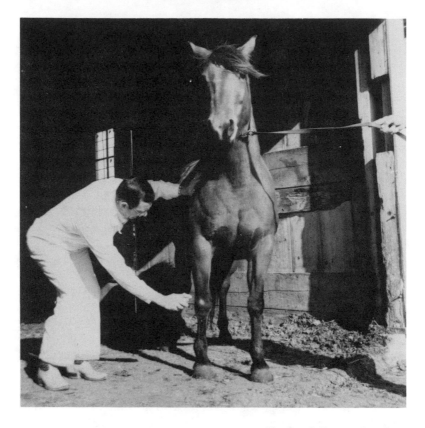

*Norden Laboratories, Inc.*
A large animal veterinarian doctors a backyard pleasure equine.

at the hospital, sale barn, or ranch. Treating an animal in the field is much more challenging. Ingenuity and cowboy ability are required when the only means of restraint available is a rope and a fence post. Beef cattle raised on a huge Wyoming ranch may have never seen a human, let alone been touched by one. Treatment of these semiwild creatures can develop into a romp 'em, stomp 'em flurry of horns and hooves. Completely opposite is the hand-reared 4-H heifer, an animal raised with close human contact and almost petlike in behavior.

Sheep and goats are slightly easier to handle because of their

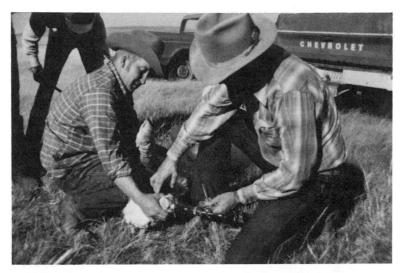

*Norden Laboratories, Inc.*
Cowboy abilities are required of a veterinarian in treating an animal in
the field.

smaller size. Ovine (sheep) and caprine (goat) ailments are similar
to those of cattle. Goats are rapidly gaining popularity as backyard
pets as people become appreciative of their affectionate and play-
ful personalities. Their small size makes them desirable for urbanites as well as families who try to be self-sufficient on a few acres.
They produce more milk than cows proportionate to their size.
They can provide a source of hypoallergenic milk for children who
are sensitive to cow's milk. Their milk is richer and higher in milk
fat than cow's milk, making delicious ice cream!

Young pigs also are relatively easy to handle, while adult
sows (female hogs) are generally confined in farrowing pens. The
most common procedures performed in porcine (pig) medicine are
castration, farrowing (birthing) assistance, vaccination, and treatment of various infections.

For the average country veterinarian, poultry comprises a small
percentage of the caseload. The large poultry and egg producers
use veterinarians who are poultry specialists and travel across the
country serving their clients. A poultry producer with hundreds of

thousands of birds cannot rely on a local large animal practitioner. Bird diseases tend to spread rapidly and can wipe out an entire flock in a matter of weeks. For small farms with only a few birds, it is generally uneconomical to call a veterinarian.

Special mention should be made of women who wish to deal with large animals. There is absolutely no reason why a member of the "weaker sex" cannot become an excellent large animal veterinarian, with one qualification. She must have a high level of self-confidence. Seldom will a woman receive the initial acceptance that a male veterinarian would receive. She must "prove" herself.

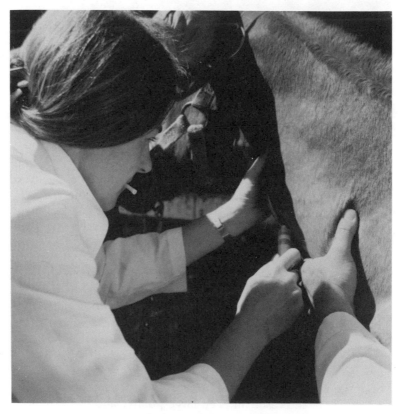

*Norden Laboratories, Inc.*
A female veterinarian treats a large animal with full competence.

She must have a tremendous amount of self-esteem in combination with her medical expertise if she is to acquire the clients' trust. Horse owners are more willing to welcome a woman; livestock owners may be more reserved. Some farmers are even reluctant to discuss their cow's "female problems" with a woman veterinarian. Any female considering a career as a large animal veterinarian should *definitely* acquire experience working with livestock or horses during high school or college. Just having her own backyard horse is not sufficient. In summary, a woman should not hesitate to pursue a goal of working with farm animals as long as she can project a confident image and can endure whatever weather Mother Nature sees fit to send. After all, a 210-pound man can no more control a 2,000-pound bull than can a 115-pound woman!

Similarly, students from an urban background should not hesitate to pursue a career in large animal medicine. Most large animal practitioners come from a rural environment, but many "city kids" decide while in veterinary school that horses or livestock are their primary interest. A special understanding is required to handle large animals effectively, an understanding that stems from experience. While young veterinarians who have been raised on a farm may have an initial advantage, city dwellers can gain the experience and confidence necessary to work with large animals.

Currently in large animal medicine a major emphasis is being placed on herd health care. The veterinarian's role is to advise the rancher or dairyman on how to keep the herd healthy. The money spent on preventive medicine for the entire herd (worming, vaccinations, estrus detection, adequate nutrition, sanitary environment) is less than the cost of treating individual illnesses and injuries. The animal producer is in business to make a profit. That profit can be maximized by incorporating the veterinarian in his overall plans. No longer is the large animal practitioner limited to the treatment of sick animals (often nicknamed "fire engine medicine"). He should be considered a partner in the agricultural business.

The small family farm with diverse types of livestock is becoming almost obsolete, primarily because it is not economically efficient. Taking its place are larger, more efficient livestock units that specialize in one breed of animal. Thousands of steers are fed in enormous feedlots. Similar numbers of hogs can be raised at a single facility. Less time and less work are involved per animal thanks to innovations. Livestock production methods must have added efficiency to counterbalance a narrow profit margin. To be of assistance, the veterinarian needs to know how much it costs to feed a steer to market weight, or the farmer's expense to produce a gallon of milk, or how much money is lost keeping a sow with a reproductive disorder.

The American livestock producer is the most productive of any in the world. This could never have been accomplished without a competent veterinary profession to lend support. Practitioners not only assist individual producers but also serve on agricultural committees and other interest groups to help promote American agriculture. Veterinarians are, in a very real, very large way, responsible for America's ability to feed the world.

## Mixed Animal Practitioner

The mixed (or general) animal veterinarian has the best and the worst of both worlds. He is generally a courageous person who is willing to tackle any situation. As a rule, he accepts any species of animal from turtle to peacock to llama. Diversification is his way of life.

In some ways, however, the practice is not as difficult as it may seem at first. The veterinarian's education was designed to provide a solid basis for the medical treatment of all animals. Although anatomy and physiology may vary somewhat between species of animals, once the principles of medicine are mastered they can be applied to canaries as well as turkeys, ponies as well as Clydesdales.

Rare is the mixed animal veterinarian who can afford the time and energy to excel in any one specialty. He is virtually a "jack of all trades." Keeping current on new techniques and drugs for cats, dogs, horses, pigs, goats, cows, and you-name-it is a formidable task. Yet even with these diverse responsibilities, the average mixed animal veterinarian earns less than either the small or large animal practitioner. His average salary (before taxes) is $35,000.

Approximately 40 percent of the 35,000 private practice veterinarians are engaged in mixed practice. The mixed animal practitioner is typically located in a small town or rural area. He divides his days between the clinic and the road. He may castrate thirty baby pigs and carry back to the clinic the sweet scent of hog manure. No wonder the owner of "Snookums," the toy poodle, wrinkles her nose when the veterinarian enters the examination room.

Mixed animal practitioners seem to spend most of their day in a hurry, rushing from farm to farm to clinic. The speed at which a country veterinarian moves is illustrated by the story of a veterinarian who was flying to a convention. After a meal had been served, his seatmate commented, "You certainly made quick work of your dinner. You must be a vet with a mixed practice."

## COMPARISON OF VETERINARY SALARIES

| Type of Employment | 1986 Average Starting Salary | 1985 Mean Income |
|---|---|---|
| Large animal | $21,900 | $43,481 |
| Mixed animal | $20,487 | $43,329 |
| Small animal | $21,620 | $49,098 |
| University | $15,833 | $43,604 |
| Federal government | $23,500 | $43,323 |
| Military service | $25,736 | $41,688 |
| State/local government | $28,560 | $40,549 |
| Industry/commercial | $28,500 | $62,547 |

*Sources:* "Employment, Starting Salaries, and Educational Indebtedness of 1986 Graduates of US Veterinary Medical Colleges," *Journal of the American Veterinary Medical Association*, January 15, 1987, Vol. 190, No.2, p.209; "1985 Incomes of US Veterinarians," *Journal of the American Veterinary Medical Association*, May 15, 1987, Vol. 190, No.10, p.1333.

# Chapter IV

# Government and Public Health Careers

Since three quarters of all veterinarians are in private practice, that leaves approximately 10,000 who are employed by either the government or private industry. Because of a predicted excess of private practice veterinarians, many veterinary colleges are encouraging students to pursue employment in areas other than clinical medicine. The United States government employs more than 3,200 veterinarians, making it the largest employer. The Department of Agriculture (USDA) employs more veterinarians than any other single agency, but veterinarians are needed in areas as diverse as the Fish and Wildlife Service, the Centers for Disease Control, the Food and Drug Administration, and the National Aeronautics and Space Administration.

Many of these government employees are engaged in what is known as regulatory medicine. Their two main goals are to control or eliminate livestock disease and to protect the public from animal diseases that can affect people.

These regulatory veterinarians inspect and quarantine animals brought into the United States from other countries to prevent the introduction of foreign diseases. Livestock diseases such as foot-and-mouth disease, contagious pleuropneumonia, and rinderpest have been kept outside the continental limits of the U.S. through the vigilance of federal regulatory veterinarians. Other diseases such as brucellosis, tuberculosis, hog cholera, screwworm, and anthrax, which previously cost millions of dollars in annual losses in the U.S., have been nearly or entirely eradicated.

The quarantining of animals is particularly necessary in an age when global transportation is so common and so fast. In less than a day a diseased animal can be flown halfway around the world. The disease can spread like wildfire in countries whose animals have not previously been exposed to it and therefore have no immunity. Birds are particularly notorious for spreading exotic diseases. Inspection and quarantine are made not only of animals, but also meat and animal by-products used in items such as clothing, leather, feed, medicine, and fertilizer.

Two of the above-mentioned diseases are transmissible to man and represent significant public health problems. Brucellosis can infect humans who handle tissues, drink unpasteurized milk, or consume improperly cooked meat from infected animals. Tuberculosis is transmissible to humans in unpasteurized milk from infected cows and goats. Both diseases are most prevalent among livestock owners, veterinarians, and workers in meat processing and rendering plants. They are "reportable diseases"; the veterinarian is required to inform the government of any case he finds. The government has instituted a testing program whereby animals infected with either disease are identified and marked for slaughter. Owners of condemned cattle are partially compensated for their loss by indemnity payments from state and federal governments. This "test and slaughter" program is necessary for two reasons: (1) it helps prevent disease in man; and (2) it helps prevent millions of dollars in losses to the livestock industry.

Brucellosis and tuberculosis are only two of the diseases that federal veterinarians are trying to eradicate. Many have already been successfully controlled. The U.S. government was responsible for developing an ingenious method of controlling screwworms, the larvae of the fly *Cochliomyia hominivorax*. In the United States they are found mainly in the Southern states. The fly lays 200 to 400 eggs on the edges of skin wounds of animals. These eggs hatch into larvae, or screwworms. At one time screwworms caused losses up to $100 million dollars to the livestock industry as a result of complications from hemorrhage, absorption of toxins, or secondary infections.

In 1958 federal veterinarians devised an imaginative yet effective method to eradicate screwworms. The key to the plan was that the female fly breeds only once in a lifetime. The veterinarians raised screwworms in captivity, exposed them to radiation that caused sterility, and released them in sufficient quantity to outnumber the native flies. When the females bred with sterile males, no offspring were produced. Since the program was begun the number of native flies has diminished to the point that very few fertile matings occur. Screwworm infestation has decreased to such a low level that if a veterinarian or rancher suspects screwworms in his livestock he should immediately report it to regulatory officials. However, permanent elimination of screwworms from the U.S. cannot be achieved until they are eradicated in Mexico.

The success of the screwworm eradication program is not attributable only to the federal and state agencies involved. Thousands of livestock producers contributed time and money to the effort. This victory in animal disease control is an example of what private citizens and government agencies can do in cooperation.

Veterinarians in the Food Safety and Inspection Service of the USDA oversee meat, poultry, and dairy inspections. The meat inspections cover cattle, sheep, goats, swine, fish, poultry, and horses (as used in pet foods) both before and after slaughter. These veterinarians supervise the preparation of meat products, including making sure the labeling is accurate and not false or misleading. They guard against harmful preservatives. They are responsible for checking food for dangerous residues such as hormones, pesticides, and antibiotics.

Veterinarians in the Food and Drug Administration are responsible for inspection of pharmaceutical (drug) and biological (vaccine) production facilities. All drugs are tested for safety and to assure that they do what the manufacturer claims they do. The same is true of feed additives used in livestock feed to help promote growth. Federal veterinarians make sure that no residues of livestock drugs or feed additives pass in meat or dairy products to people.

The U.S. government also sponsors many areas of research. It has a multimillion-dollar budget for veterinary research. Sometimes grants are provided to veterinary colleges. In other cases the government supplies the funding, personnel, and facilities required to solve problems of current importance. Federal veterinarians are constantly engaged in research for new methods of control for viruses, bacteria, fungi, and parasites. They also con-

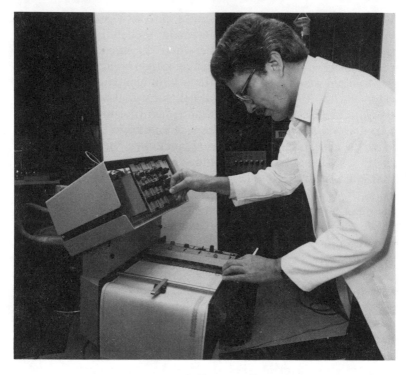

*University of Illinois College of Veterinary Medicine*
A researcher studies data.

duct studies on noninfectious problems such as bloat in cattle and the effects of pesticides. One vital area where more knowledge is needed is the effects of nuclear fallout and radiation in livestock and therefore humans.

One predicament being faced by governments around the world is a serious, yet almost comical, situation, the prevalence of methane gas. Ruminants are animals with four stomachs which, thanks to microbes that live in those stomachs, can readily digest grass and other plants. Cows, sheep, and goats are examples of ruminants. As a by-product of the ruminant's digestive system, methane is produced. It is similar to the gas that is produced by people, particularly when they eat something that doesn't agree with them. As everyone knows, when a person or an animal "passes gas," the odor is unpleasant. Ruminants are very efficient methane producers, releasing copious amounts of the malodorous gas into the atmosphere every day. It has been estimated that one sheep produces five gallons of methane daily.

Far from being a joke, this pollutant is a contributor to a potentially serious environmental hazard. The concentration of methane 30,000 years ago was only a third what it is today. Scientists fear that these high levels of methane contribute to the phenomenon known as the greenhouse effect, which could cause a dangerous rise in the earth's temperatures and even a melting of the polar ice caps. Governments around the world need to work together to minimize methane production from all sources, including animals.

The United States government functions on the local level in some states through Extension veterinarians. The groundwork for extension veterinarians was laid in 1862 by the Morrill Act, which created the land-grant university system. The Act enabled agriculture to take a prominent position in American higher education. The Smith-Lever Act of 1914 established the Cooperative Extension Service as a cooperative between state and local governments in partnership with the U.S. Department of Agriculture, state land-grant colleges and universities, and county government. These educational and political institutions jointly fund and guide the Extension Service in its dissemination of research and educational information.

Extension veterinarians are specialists in the Extension system. Their function is multifaceted. They interpret, disseminate, and encourage practical use of knowledge in veterinary medicine among other veterinarians, regulatory officials, and county extension personnel. They also act as a liaison between veterinary colleges and livestock organizations, livestock producers, and animal owners. They interpret the results obtained through research and relay these findings to people and organizations who can put them to practical use—private practice veterinarians, private industry and commercial concerns, and livestock producers. Extension veterinarians disseminate information about new products, preferred practices, and implementation of new laws and regulations through the mass media, public meetings, demonstration projects, personal visits, newsletters, continuing education programs, computers, livestock organizations, and youth programs.

Their major emphasis is on food animals, but they also deal with horses and small animals. The Extension Service has been a valuable adjunct to animal disease control and eradication programs such as those dealing with tuberculosis, hog cholera, cattle scabies, Newcastle disease, and brucellosis. Extension veterinarians have contributed to the most plentiful, reasonably priced, safe, and wholesome food supply in the world.

There are approximately 125 Extension veterinarians, some employed full time, others part time. The majority have advanced degrees or are Board-certified. As members of the academic community, they must have a high degree of intellectual ability. Through written, spoken, and visual skills they must be able to communicate and work well with people. Teaching ability is a must. Some Extension veterinarians are involved with research, whereas others concentrate on clinical teaching and diagnostic service programs. As in so many other areas, future Extension veterinarians will become involved in computer software development and data transmission.

The Fish and Wildlife Service is a branch of the U.S. Department of Interior and employs veterinarians for several purposes. The National Wildlife Health Center, for example, deals with research and diagnosis of wildlife diseases. Another responsibility of veterinarians in the Fish and Wildlife Service is to help control zoonotic disease (diseases that are transmissible from animals to man or vice versa.) Diseases such as leptospirosis, tularemia, and tapeworms are a few such diseases that can pass from wild animals to humans. In another branch of the Fish and Wildlife Service veterinarians investigate the natural habitat, nutrition, and reproduction of wild animals in order to save these species threatened by continual human expansion. Veterinarians also do extensive research on the captive propagation of endangered species.

The Canadian Department of Agriculture operates on principles similar to that of the Unites States. The Food Production and Inspection Branch is responsible for meat hygiene, livestock inspection, research into disease control, and extension services.

Although the federal government is the largest employer of veterinarians, many jobs also exist with state and local governments. Each state has a veterinarian, usually operating in the state Department of Agriculture, whose duties are to look after the health of animals by enforcing the laws and regulations drawn for that purpose. In many states the state veterinarian has a corps of assistant veterinarians. As one of their responsibilities, state veterinarians control the movement of disease into and within the state. Animals cannot be transported across state lines without veterinary inspection and a permit. Hawaii is particularly strict, since rabies is not present anywhere on the islands; all animals, including vaccinated pets, must undergo a six-month quarantine before they are allowed into the state. State health departments also hire veterinarians to help control animal diseases transmissible to man (for example, rabies), as well as handle meat and poultry inspection. Canadian provinces operate similarly to protect the health of their citizens and animals.

Some cities have full- or part-time veterinarians as members of their health department. They investigate disease outbreaks such as food poisoning, ringworm, or plague. They evaluate the safety of food processing plants and water supplies. They study and investigate the effects of various pesticides, industrial pollutants, and other sources of contamination. Large metropolitan areas have tax-supported animal shelters for stray and homeless animals, many of which employ veterinarians full or part time.

The advantages of government employment are well known to any veterinarian in private practice. A forty-hour workweek, pleasant working conditions and environment, paid vacations and holidays, and job security can greatly reduce the level of stress in a veterinarian's life. A reasonable salary accompanies these jobs. An average salary for a veterinarian employed by the U.S. or state government is $40,000, considerably more than a veterinarian earns in the early years of private practice. On the other hand, the government imposes limitations on the maximum amount any employee can earn, so the potential income for private practice veterinarians is much higher.

*Chapter* **V**

# Military Careers

The military division of the federal government also employs veterinarians in the U.S. Army Veterinary Corps (one of six separate corps comprising the Army Medical Department) and in the Air Force. Previously, the military veterinarian's main responsibility was the military horses. Today, although a few military horses still exist, veterinary officers are involved in health care and the selection, training, and health of sentry dogs, laboratory animals, and animals used in space travel. They also treat the pets of military personnel.

At military installations, the veterinarians are responsible for the preservation of human health. They are responsible for food hygiene, safety, wholesomeness, and quality assurance to safeguard the health of military personnel. Their inspections also protect the interests of the government with respect to contract specifications.

The responsibilities of military veterinarians are not limited to the United States. Around the world they raise the standards of animal production, improve food processing and distribution, and control animal diseases transmissible to man. Sanitation, handling of food and water supplies, waste disposal, and insect and rodent control all come under the jurisdiction of the overseas military veterinarian.

Many veterinary officers, both abroad and in the states, are engaged in biomedical research. For instance, Air Force veterinarians are responsible for space and conventional flight projects. They study the biomedical reaction to space travel and develop nutrition programs for space flights. Approximately one-third of the military veterinarians are engaged in research of some kind.

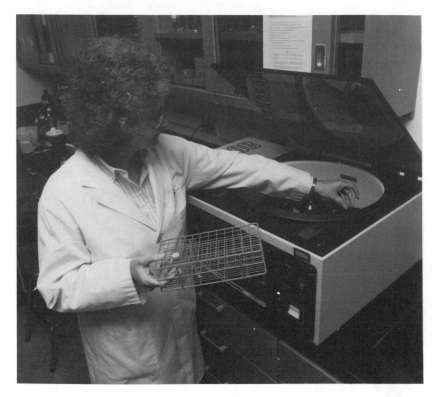

*University of Illinois College of Veterinary Medicine*
Preparation of samples.

Many of them have advanced degrees in pathology, physiology, microbiology, toxicology, and public health to enable them to carry out and evaluate their research.

Physically qualified graduates of veterinary schools may apply for appointment in military service, with the grade being determined by the age, professional experience, and qualifications of the applicant. The United States military demands professional excellence of its veterinarians. Over 40 percent of the military career veterinarians are board-certified in specialty branches of veterinary medicine. The military offers veterinary students financial assistance for their education in exchange for later service in the armed forces.

The average military veterinarian's salary in the mid-1980's was $40,000. Benefits such as medical services for the officer and his family, PX privileges, pension, and travel opportunities are added bonuses to the veterinarian's compensation. The military veterinarian can enjoy early retirement at half pay and still be young enough to enjoy a second career.

# Chapter VI

# Private Industry Careers

As was mentioned previously, concern exists about a potential overabundance of veterinarians in private practice within the next ten years. As a result, a growing number of veterinarians are finding employment with private companies. These persons acquire specialized training in nutrition, virology, pharmacology, microbiology, bacteriology, toxicology, parasitology, and other fields that enables them to carry out the clinical evaluation necessary for developing new products.

Many kinds of companies hire veterinarians. Biological and pharmaceutical companies need them to oversee laboratory animals and to develop new and improved vaccines and drugs. Both human and veterinary pharmaceutical companies employ veterinarians. Many years of testing and hundreds of thousands of dollars are required before the Federal Drug Administration allows a drug (even an animal drug) to go on the market. Some human drugs (such as hormones) are actually animal by-products. For instance, the insulin a diabetic injects comes from an animal's pancreas. Besides biological and pharmaceutical companies, scientific instrument manufacturers conduct research to devise better products. Veterinarians are also needed in the marketing and sale of the products these companies manufacture.

Companies that manufacture animal feeds employ a large number of veterinarians. The livestock industry is based on dollars and cents; livestock producers view animals as a business. The beef industry is an excellent example. To maximize profits, producers try to minimize the time required to raise a steer from birth to slaughter. Every day longer required to reach market weight means less income for the rancher, the feedlot, etc. Feed companies determine the optimal feed ingredients needed to maximize gain. They also add growth stimulants, parasiticides, and antibiotics to the feed. If a steer contracts a respiratory infection or worms, his development will be set back weeks, which is costly to the producer. Veterinarians are employed to determine the economic feasibility of these added ingredients. Do they result in enough weight gain to justify their cost? Also, veterinarians determine whether residues from these additives remain in the meat, potentially resulting in a public health problem.

The same idea lies behind all animal feed. Dairymen want the

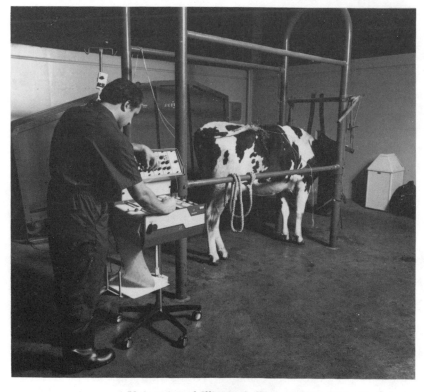

*University of Illinois College of Veterinary Medicine*
Physical readings are being taken from this cow as part of a research project.

maximum amount of milk from their cows. They know that nutrition plays an essential role in milk production, and they turn to the feed company (and the company's veterinarian) for help. Sheep ranchers want abundant meat and wool. Horse owners (both pleasure horses and racehorses) are interested in maximum nutrition and disease control. The veterinary nutritionist realizes that with increased production (milk in a dairy cow, mutton in a sheep, or speed in a horse) comes an increased demand for vitamins, minerals, protein, and carbohydrates.

Pet food is also included in this category. Many special diets have been developed for various phases of pet health. For instance, puppies, kittens, and nursing mothers require diets high in energy, protein, calcium, and phosphorus. Special diets have been formulated for cats with potentially fatal urinary problems. Many older animals suffer from kidney and heart disease; diets low in protein, salt, and minerals help these animals live longer, more enjoyable lives. Foods are being developed to help prevent bone and joint disease in large breeds of dog.

Besides the development of new pharmaceutical and feed products, private companies employ veterinarians for other reasons. Meat packing plants need veterinarians to ensure quality control. Some veterinarians with a journalistic flair work with publishing houses writing books and articles on various phases of veterinary medicine. Other private businesses that hire full- or part-time veterinarians are racetracks, brood mare farms, zoos, circuses, aquariums, fur ranches, large livestock breeding enterprises, and humane societies.

Across the United States, many cities have humane societies and Societies for the Prevention of Cruelty to Animals. Many of these are nonprofit and are privately operated (not city or county funded). The larger ones in metropolitan areas employ one or more veterinarians full time. Smaller societies hire local veterinarians on a part-time contract basis. They are responsible for the thousands of homeless and stray animals that pass through the shelters annually. Some animals are injured, and the veterinarian must decide which ones should be treated and which should be humanely destroyed. The majority of the societies make certain that dogs and cats are spayed or castrated before being adopted into new homes.

Humane societies also rescue exotic animals, such as alligators, ocelots, snakes, and skunks from trees, sewers, and backyards. Typically, the owners of these animals once thought they would make good pets but soon tired of them. By and large, exotic animals do not make satisfactory pets.

Keeping disease under control in a shelter full of homeless unvaccinated animals, many of whom are in poor nutrition, is a major challenge for the humane society veterinarian. When a new owner adopts a puppy or a kitten, he expects it to be healthy. Yet viruses and bacteria can spread throughout a shelter population within forty-eight hours. Teaching sanitation methods to shelter personnel is a priority of the veterinarian.

For a veterinarian with altruistic values, a humane society career can be tremendously rewarding and satisifying. The veterinarian knows he can use his skills to help defenseless animals and directly minimize animal suffering.

But the job offers heart-wrenching situations also. Some animals have been abused, starved, or tortured by their previous owners. Neglect and irresponsibility are even greater problems. Irresponsible pet owners allow too many dogs and cats to breed and produce offspring. Cats are so prolific that one female can result in 7,822 offspring in her lifetime (including her offspring's offspring, etc.). For an adult dog or cat in an animal shelter, the odds favor its being euthanized (put to sleep) rather than finding a loving home. Annually, 15 million stray dogs and cats are euthanized by shelters, humane societies, dog pounds, and so on. Another 60 million strays meet violent death (starvation, hit by a car, shot). The way a so-called civilized society treats the animals that is has domesticated should disgust any decent, caring person.

The benefits and drawbacks of working for private industry are similar to those of the government. Benefits include good hours, pleasant working conditions, paid vacations, retirement plans, paid insurance, and fringe benefits. These are counterbalanced by salaries which, although generally very good, are confined to preset limits. Surveys conducted in the mid-1980's show that new graduates in private industry earn annual salaries of less than $35,000. Experienced veterinarians average $65,000 annually.

*Chapter* **VII**

# Zoo Veterinarians

Mention should be made of zoo veterinarians as a specialty group. Every major U.S. zoological garden (including marine exhibits such as Sea World) has at least one full-time veterinarian on staff. However, only about 125 veterinarians earn their living exclusively through zoo employment. Many of the smaller zoos have working arrangements with local veterinarians who want to diversify their practice with exotic animal medicine.

The daily routine of the zoo veterinarian includes treating injuries and illnesses. An animal may develop gastrointestinal problems from feeding by zoo visitors. The veterinarian may be called to assist an animal who is having trouble giving birth. Broken bones occur in zoo animals just as in domestic animals. In addition to treatment and surgery, a large portion of a veterinarian's day is devoted to preventive medicine, that is, keeping the animals healthy. Preventive medicine for captive wild animals is very similar to that for pets and farm animals. Teeth need to be floated, nails and hooves trimmed, and animals vaccinated and wormed.

Working with zoos does not involve just day-to-day medicine such as extracting a tiger's tooth or doctoring a wound in a flamingo or vaccinating wolves. It also involves a commitment to the long-term health and well-being of all zoo animals. It is the duty of the zoo (and therefore the zoo veterinarian) to make the animal's life resemble, as closely as possible, a normal existence in the wild. Only then can the animal lead a pleasant life. The change from a free living environment to confinement is a source of potential problems in these captive animals, and veterinarians must find ways to deal with them. Research continues into the nutritional needs of zoo animals. Many animals reproduce poorly in captivity,

69

while others are so prolific that they need to be placed on birth control drugs. The zoo veterinarian needs day-to-day medical skills as well as long-term vision.

Zoo veterinarians are intensely interested in the preservation of all animal species. Remarkable advances have been made in keeping endangered species from becoming extinct. In fact, some species (such as the Amoy tiger, European bison, Pere David's deer, and Przewalski horse) can no longer be found in the wild and exist only in zoos. Thanks to man's encroachment on their territory, these animals had almost disappeared. Through the efforts of zoos, they were preserved and have been successfully propagated in captivity. Zoological gardens also strive to reestablish vanishing species in their natural habitat. Zoos have succeeded in reintroducing into nature the American bison, the Golden Lion marmoset, and the Nene goose (the state bird of Hawaii).

Zoo veterinarians also engage in scientific research. Veterinarians can then use the results of their previous research to monitor the animals' gene pool. They are able to breed desirable characteristics into offspring by knowing the inheritable characteristics of the parents and the composition of their genes and chromosomes. Veterinarians can freeze semen and ova for later use. The semen from a snow leopard in New York may be used to impregnate a female snow leopard in California if veterinarians feel the union will produce hardier, more desirable offspring.

Zoo veterinarians have also achieved several interspecies embryo transfers. For example, a zebra embryo was placed in the uterus of a horse and carried full term to successful birth. The same procedure was used with a domestic Holstein cow acting as a surrogate mother to a gaur (a breed of East Indian wild ox).

In addition to practicing medicine and performing research, zoo veterinarians have other responsibilities. They handle food inspection for the animals, they help plan exhibits and displays, and they aid in the education of the public and of the zoo personnel. Some veterinarians also serve as zoo directors.

Veterinary schools offer relatively little in the direct field of exotic animal medicine. The veterinarian's education is designed to provide a foundation upon which to build. Once the basic principles of medicine are learned, they can be applied to individual species. The veterinarian uses the same medical concepts to treat an antelope as he would use to treat an Angus cow. The main differences lie not in the illnesses but rather in the restraint and anesthesia used. That is where exotic animal medicine offers its unique challenges.

One educational possibility for students interested in zoo medicine is a preceptorship of one or two months' duration at a zoo before graduation. After graduation, internships and residencies are available at large zoos, such as that in San Diego, and at a few veterinary schools.

# Chapter VIII

# Educational Careers

The academically oriented veterinarian may find his haven in teaching. The United States and Canada have thirty-one colleges of veterinary medicine, each of which has between 50 and 150 veterinarians on staff. The veterinarian who decides to go into teaching typically engages in private practice for a while before rcentering the academic world. It would be difficult to teach a subject without having any "real life" experience.

A veterinary professor must have a special interest in or devotion to a particular field of medicine, such as microbiology or small animal surgery. He must have a master's degree or be willing to obtain one within a couple of years. Some have a doctorate. Many veterinary educators are board-certified in their area of expertise.

The responsibilities of a veterinarian employed at a veterinary college are threefold: (1) teaching; (2) research; and (3) clinical medicine.

Obviously, the primary concern of a veterinary educator should be teaching. The professor should truly enjoy dealing with students, both lecturing to them as a group and working with them one-on-one. He should be good communicator, both in the written and the spoken language.

Veterinary professors are so knowledgeable in their chosen subject material that they are usually limited to teaching one or two courses at the most. During the students' first two years of veterinary school, their professors teach classroom studies such as developmental anatomy, parasitology, or virology. During the last two years the professors help the students apply their learning to clinical situations. A professor in a veterinary clinic may teach students applied respiratory physiology, neurology, or avian medicine.

If a veterinary educator only teaches only one or two courses, what does he do the rest of the time? The remainder of his time involves his second responsibility—research. In addition to teaching, he is expected to do research in his particular area of interest and publish his findings in veterinary journals. Research can be conducted in laboratories, such as ascertaining the half-life of drugs in animals; or it can take place in fields or barns, such as synchronizing the reproductive cycles of dairy goats under true-to-life conditions. Major advances in veterinary medicine often come from universities.

Veterinary colleges receive funding from many sources besides student tuition and state tax money. Usually research money comes from these other sources. The federal government, private companies, and animal welfare groups all contribute to veterinary colleges for research in animal health problems. For example, a pharmaceutical company may contribute hundreds of thousands of dollars for university research into the feline urological syndrome. A wealthy person whose cat died of feline leukemia may donate a similar sum with the stipulation that it be spent on research into that disease.

An example of research currently being done at universities are the experiments being conducted to eliminate salmonella food poisoning in humans. The *Salmonella* bacterium is found in unsanitary meat and poultry products. When humans eat such contaminated food, they experience fever, headache, nausea, and diarrhea. Severe cases can result in death. In laboratory tests, researchers have genetically altered the bacterium by deleting two of its genes. It is thus rendered harmless but is capable of provoking a protective response from the body's immune system. The hope is that this genetically engineered microbe can be used to vaccinate farm animals. If livestock and poultry can resist *Salmonella*, their meat cannot carry the bacterium to people. After further tests at the university level, the concept will probably go to private industry for development, testing, licensing, and manufacturing.

In addition to teaching and research, the veterinarian who chooses to be a clinician at a veterinary college also treats animals.

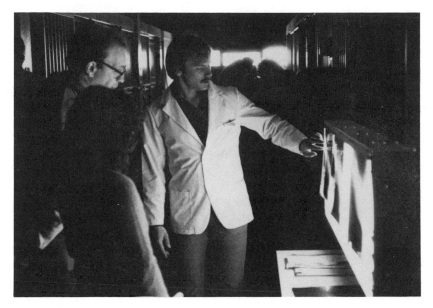

*University of Illinois College of Veterinary Medicine*
Veterinary Medicine Open House gives this student an opportunity to explain X-rays to college visitors.

He doctors animals brought into the college's veterinary hospital just as a veterinarian does in private practice. Not only must he excel in his medical field, but he must be capable of good client relations. Veterinarians in private practice can refer difficult cases to the veterinary college, knowing that experts (veterinary cardiologists, ophthalmologists, equine practitioners, surgeons) will give the animal the best possible treatment. University veterinary hospitals are better equipped than most private ones.

Good veterinary instructors are in demand, and it is easy to see why. They must have years of post-D.V.M. education. They must have an intense interest in one specialized branch of veterinary medicine. They must be competent to use the thousands of dollars earmarked for their research. They must be capable of publishing their findings. They must enjoy students. They must be good communicators. They must be both medically and socially oriented. And here's the real clincher. This person who is expected to excel in so many different fields is paid only average wages for a veterinarian.

Typical salaries of veterinarians working at colleges or universities are $40,000 to $45,000. Academic positions progress up the scale from instructor to assistant professor to professor to department head to dean.

Although 75 percent of veterinarians involved in educational programs are employed at veterinary schools, the positions are also available with human medical colleges in their laboratory animal departments. Also, veterinarians are needed to teach students who want to be veterinary technicians.

# Chapter IX

# Alternative Careers in Veterinary Medicine

Within the categories previously discussed are unlimited subclassifications. In fact, veterinary colleges are encouraging students to pursue less conventional careers in veterinary medicine because of the increasing competition in clinical medicine.

The competition facing private practices stems from several sources. First, increasing numbers of practitioners are graduating from school. For years most veterinary schools consistently increased their class size. The prediction in the 1960's and 1970's was for an insufficient number of veterinarians to meet the needs of the last two decades of the century. Now that prediction has been reversed: an excess of graduate veterinarians is foreseen within the next decade. Currently several schools are decreasing the number of students accepted for each class. Nevertheless, veterinary schools produce many more new graduates then they did twenty-five years ago. Estimates place the number of veterinarians in private practice at 40,000 by 1990, an increase of 14 percent over 1987.

Many veterinarians are entering unconventional branches of private practice, such as mobile clinics, low-cost spay clinics, vaccination clinics, and tax-exempt government-subsidized animal welfare groups. Some veterinarians feel that advertising (television, direct mail, newspapers, Yellow Pages ads) is necessary to maintain their business. The veterinarians with these novel ideas are in direct competition with the conventional practitioner. To further complicate the situation, many observers are projecting growth in consumer demand for veterinary services, but slower growth than in the last few decades. Many economists predict that the supply of practitioners will far outdistance the demand for their services.

In addition to increasing numbers of veterinarians, feed stores and pet health centers also compete with private practitioners for over-the-counter drug sales. Livestock and horse owners commonly purchase drugs from their local agricultural co-op or feed store, and the same is true of pet owners and pet stores. The employees at these stores are more than willing to give free advice on use of these drugs and animal health products.

How will new graduates earn a living in a society that is already saturated with animal doctors as well as the quasi-veterinarians? Tomorrow's veterinarian will need to be open-minded toward a variety of outlets for his professional talents.

As one solution, more and more small animal veterinarians are specializing, for instance limiting their expertise to ophthalmology, dentistry, dermatology, or surgery and relying on other veterinarians to refer difficult cases to them. These specialists are usually board-certified, having pursued advanced education and passed an extensive examination conducted by the Board of their specialty. Veterinary medicine will probably follow the example of human medicine, where specialization is not only accepted but expected by the public.

One field that has previously been neglected is small animal dentistry. Although equine dentistry has been practiced for decades, oral medicine and surgery for pets is just coming of age. The teeth and gums of dogs and cats have the same composition as their human counterparts, but animals never brush their teeth. Maybe brushing a cat's teeth sounds ridiculous, but they need brushing to maintain oral hygiene. Periodontal disease (infected gums) is now recognized as affecting more than 80 percent of dogs and cats over three years of age. Bacteria from infected gums can infiltrate the blood and be carried throughout the body, resulting in heart, liver, and kidney disease. Pets with periodontal disease must have their teeth scaled and polished or eventually lose the teeth. Besides routine cleaning, other dentistry techniques are being used in small animals. Pet owners will be hearing more about root canal, gum resection, and even orthodontia.

The emergence of pet health insurance will also provide impetus to the trend toward specialization. If the insurance company, not the owner, pays the fees for extensive treatment or surgery, more animals will receive needed medical care instead of being euthanized.

The small animal emergency clinician is a specialist in his own right. He is either employed by or owns an animal emergency clinic. Emergency clinics are becoming more and more common, especially in medium-sized and large cities. The emergency clinician must be quick-thinking as well as compassionate, since he constantly deals with injured or sick animals and distraught owners. Needless to say, the hours tend to be undesirable (nights, weekends, and holidays). Because of these features the salary for an emergency veterinarian is slightly higher than for a regular practitioner.

Believe it or not, animal psychology is a growing field. Many owners have a pet they love but one with a personality problem that makes it difficult, if not impossible, to live with. Such owners are willing to pay for advice from an expert in animal behavior. Many people do not realize how emotional stress can affect pets. A divorce in the family can cause a normally easygoing, docile dog to begin defecating on the floor or bed, chewing sores in its skin, or acting lame for sympathy. Cats in particular are prone to displaying the psychological reaction of inappropriate urination. The misconduct of dogs who display aggression, overprotection of their owner, submissive wetting, car chasing, finicky eating, fear of thunder, and coprophagia (eating feces) can be managed through proper behavior modification techniques. Usually the veterinary psychologist needs to work with both the pet and the owner.

Veterinary medicine is slow in acknowledging the potential value of chiropractic medicine in both large and small animal medicine. Veterinary schools do not include such courses in the curriculum. Graduates of chiropractic schools are licensed to practice on humans only; legally they cannot work on animals. Therefore, some veterinarians with an interest in chiropractic medicine have returned to school to obtain a chiropractic degree after receiving their D.V.M. They then apply what they have learned to animals.

Also increasing in demand is veterinary holistic medicine, which means treating not just the disease but the animal as a whole, including its environment, owner, nutrition, and psychological needs. Holistic medicine is actually a more complete approach to animal health than are the current somatic methods. Veterinary acupuncture, while far from common, is likewise gaining popularity.

Large animal medicine has its share of unique specialties. In addition to species specialization, distinctions arise within each species. Mention has already been made of the differences between a pleasure-horse and a racehorse veterinarian. Treating dairy goats raised for milk production is a far cry from treating Angora goats raised for their hair. Poultry production for broilers is nothing like rearing hens for egg-laying.

With an increasing world population, a more abundant and more economical food supply will be in demand. Many new techniques are looming on the horizon as possible methods of increasing world food production. In a procedure known as embryo transfer, an embryo from an expensive, genetically superior animal is transplanted into a less expensive, mixed-breed animal. The first animal can then be bred again, thus enabling a larger quantity of high-quality livestock. Along the same lines is superovulation, in which drugs are given to the female animal that allow it to produce many more ova (eggs) than normal and thus produce more offspring. Collecting and freezing livestock embryos is another facet of current research. Perfection of these and other techniques requires specialization. (An interesting side comment: Veterinarians specializing in embryo transfer are among the highest paid animal doctors in the world.)

American agriculture is becoming more and more diversified. For instance, farms that raise mink, catfish, crawfish, shrimp, worms, and snails are springing up across the nation. While being a veterinarian to a catfish may not sound particularly exciting, the producer of catfish depends on these animals for his livelihood. He wants someone to answer his questions regarding disease, nutrition, and reproduction. Researchers in shrimp mariculture programs say that the economic potential for the shrimp industry is massive.

Some veterinarians prefer relief work rather than working in just one practice. They substitute for veterinarians who are sick or on vacation. Relief work provides for a wide variety of experience, since every practice, like every household, is different. It offers the veterinarian the opportunity to work as many hours a week as he desires (a useful option for someone who wants part-time employment.) The relief veterinarian need not work in only one locale. He has the option of spending summers in New England and winters in Florida, if he desires. These veterinarians are governed by the usual licensing requirements and can practice only in states where they have a current license.

The computer age has not left veterinary medicine untouched. Veterinary hospitals are already using computers to help with bookkeeping and record-keeping. Improved software is constantly being developed. Veterinarians look forward to computer-assisted diagnosis, which involves feeding symptoms into the computer and retrieving a list of possible diagnoses. When available it will help decipher difficult cases, give advice on laboratory tests to run, evaluate the results, suggest treatment, and then modify that treatment protocol as necessary. The computer should, in theory, minimize veterinarian errors. For instance, it could detect dangerous drug interactions from improper prescriptions. Computer-assisted diagnosis is in its infancy. The goal is for clinics across the nation to tie their modems into a centralized databank that has the latest in diagnostic and treatment information. Developing such computer programs requires input from resourceful veterinarians.

Veterinarians may also choose to specialize in practice management. A veterinarian who owns his own practice spends about half his time and energy on nonmedical activities. He must be business manager, personnel director, auditor, and purchasing agent. He must devise a way of making financial ends meet. He must pay his employees adequately (but not more than the clinic can afford). He must pay himself adequately (but not so much that it drains the practice). He must charge high enough fees to generate sufficient income to pay his bills (but not so high that his clients find another veterinarian). The owner-veterinarian must keep track of payroll records, income tax withholding, unemployment compensation, and worker's compensation insurance. He must learn inventory control so that he has enough drugs on hand but not excessive capital tied up in inventory. Few veterinarians are trained to handle these responsibilities. One who has a flair for business management may serve as a consultant to other veterinarians, enabling them to have more efficient and productive practices. Several veterinarians currently travel around the United States helping individual clinics.

An interesting option for veterinarians is to combine their profession with world travel. International organizations such as the Peace Corps, the World Health Organization, and the United Nations are in need of veterinarians to implement overseas programs.

Much of the world has insufficient sources of animal protein. Some 500 to 800 million people live on the verge of hunger and malnutrition. The leaders of such nations are striving to achieve standards similar to the United States both in livestock production and human health. By teaching local farmers how to increase livestock health and production, veterinarians can make an impact on reducing world hunger. Underdeveloped countries, especially in Southeast Asia and Africa, have inadequate veterinary care, particularly preventive health care. Improving animal health may be as basic as teaching farmers about vaccination, worming for parasites, and animal nutrition.

Overseas veterinarians also strive to improve human health through proper milk and meat hygiene. Food processing procedures that seem basic to Americans (such as milk pasteurization) are novel concepts in some countries. Veterinarians develop programs to increase food sanitation and inspection in underdeveloped nations.

Serving humanity and animals overseas can be quite fulfilling emotionally while at the same time providing fascinating opportunities for travel. However, major drawbacks do exist. Foreign veterinarians face a high level of exposure to animal diseases that are contagious to man. Leptospirosis, rabies, and brucellosis are still common in underdeveloped countries. Additionally, these veterinarians must have strong, yet flexible, personalities. They must be exceptionally innovative, in good health, and adaptable to strange cultural and social traditions. They must be patient, since often the people they are trying to help cannot understand how the control of animal diseases will benefit them personally.

Another area of increasing demand is avian medicine (including pet birds, domestic fowl, and wild birds). In health-conscious America, more people are trying to lower their cholesterol levels by eating poultry instead of beef and pork. Chicken and turkey production is on the rise.

Ecologists and environmental protection groups are taking active stands for the welfare of endangered avian species. Veterinarians are needed to study and evaluate the needs of such birds both in zoos and in the wild.

Pet birds are becoming more popular, especially among apartment dwellers. Ownership of exotic birds such as cockatiels and parrots is increasing. These birds can easily cost more than a purebred dog.

In the past most veterinarians graduated from school grossly undereducated in these species. This was not entirely the schools' fault. Many students had little interest in our feathered friends. Veterinary schools are currently putting more emphasis on avian medicine.

Yet another growing area is marine biology. Eighty percent of all life on earth is found in the oceans. Marine plants and animals offer tremendous potential for increased use as food (for humans and for livestock). Veterinarians will be instrumental in the development of undersea life for the alleviation of world hunger. Considering that over 200,000 species of animals exist below the surface of the oceans, this will be no small task.

Fish are increasingly becoming victims of pollution and contamination. Toxic chemicals and nuclear by-products can easily threaten marine life. Veterinarians are needed to help avoid this disaster. Marine veterinarians are also needed to protect the public from consumption of toxic residues in fish and other aquatic animals.

Marine life is rapidly becoming a source of new drugs. Just as some medicines have been obtained from natural sources on land (such as penicillin and morphine), similar drugs are being discovered in the oceans. None are yet being marketed, but many are in the testing stage. Certain sea sponges secrete a compound that has potential for fighting the inflammation and pain of arthritis; this drug has already been tested in animals. The sea whip (a fernlike soft coral) produces a substance that has proved effective as a painkiller in animal trials. Several veterinary pharmaceutical companies are doing research on marine-based drugs, checking them for antiviral and antitumor properties. The ocean has been called the largest untapped source of new pharmaceuticals.

Veterinarians will also occupy key positions in the expanding space industry. Before man is catapulted into unexplored regions

in space, animals are used. Endless hours of preparation and experimentation go into space projects involving animals. Nutritional requirements are calculated. Body metabolism rates are
measured. The effects of space travel both on the body as a whole
and on individual cells of the body are observed. Aerospace veterinarians are employed by both private industry and the federal
government.

# Chapter X

# Psychological Profile of a Veterinarian

So after reading the preceding chapters, you're still determined to become a veterinarian, eh? You're still eager to pursue a career that combines animals and medicine. Your dream hasn't faded. This book was not written to discourage aspiring veterinarians. Rather, it was intended to present a true picture of a multifaceted profession, a picture free of romantic notions and glorified images.

So what's next? Now is the time to make an assessment of your personal characteristics and attributes. Self-evaluation cannot guarantee success, but it certainly can help in determining your happiness and potential in the profession. List your good qualities and your outstanding virtues. Also list your traits that may need some improvement, areas in which you are not quite "up to snuff." Then measure yourself against the traits that veterinarians should possess. Be honest. Remember, the perfect veterinarian does not exist any more than does the perfect person. But the following characteristics are important if you are to become a successful animal doctor, content with your choice of profession.

Veterinary medicine requires commitment. Countless times during your education you'll ask, "Is it worth it?" Only you can answer that question. You must weigh the hours of study, the effort required to achieve top grades, the expense of your education, and the potential income lost while in school. On the other side of the scale is the goal of what you hope to accomplish as a veterinarian and the satisfaction that accompanies it. Few members of our society attain the educational level of a doctor's degree (regardless of subject). Only an ambitious and highly motivated person achieves that goal.

As a student, you must get good grades. There is no way around that requirement. You should take stock of your scholastic proficiency, your organizational skills, and your ability to motivate yourself. Procrastination, poor study habits, and a lackadaisical attitude have no place in the veterinary student's life. Day after day after day of perseverance is required.

Commitment must continue after graduation through those first few frustrating years of employment. No job, career, or profession turns out to be exactly as the novice worker expects. Some unexpected and unpleasant experiences will be encountered. Mistakes (possibly costly) will be made. A formal college education does not provide the practical experience and know-how to enable the new graduate to "ooze" with self-confidence. Education continues in the work field. You must be willing to learn from your co-workers. Your new boss, fellow veterinarians, technicians, kennel workers, and even clients will have helpful information to share if you are willing to listen. The veterinarian should know what is best for the patient, take into account the wishes of the owner, and at the same time be aware of his own abilities and limitations. It takes years of experience to learn to balance and handle all those factors.

A veterinarian must have an inquisitive mind. You cannot stagnate once you receive your D.V.M. Medicine (both human and veterinary) is advancing at a faster rate than ever before. The commitment to the pursuit of knowledge must remain throughout your career. Continuing education is a must if you hope to keep abreast of your field.

That inquisitive mind should also enjoy the challenge of deciphering riddles. Making a diagnosis or pursuing an area of research and experimentation is nothing more than putting together the pieces of an intricate puzzle. Some puzzles are more difficult than others. Veterinarians are constantly presented with riddles and puzzles that are their responsibility to solve.

What else is required of a veterinarian? Obviously a humane attitude toward animals is a prerequisite. You have to truly enjoy animals. You must derive deep satisfaction from working with them. A veterinarian cannot have just an average concern for animals; he needs a sincere dedication to them. Your concern for animal welfare must be persistent and intense, not just a passing fancy.

Most animal doctors choose veterinary medicine as a career because they like animals. But take time to evaluate how much you *really* like animals. Year after year you will be working with creatures who will kick, bite, claw, and otherwise try to get the best of you. Not that the animal is necessarily malicious by nature. He simply would prefer that you leave him alone. Generally he's nervous, if not downright scared. He doesn't understand why you poked that needle into him; all he knows is that it hurt. Imagine trying your best to help a sick or injured animal who is trying his best to chew off your hand. The scenario is repeated over and over again in real life. You will see a wide range of animal dispositions. As children we are exposed to our own pets and our friends' pets, most of whom are affectionate, if not downright cuddly. A major mistake is to assume that all animals are like the ones from our childhood.

Often a humane attitude isn't enough. Compassion is a necessary attribute. For a moment, try to place yourself in the animal's position. Imagine yourself casually lounging on the porch when you are abruptly stuffed into a box with only a couple of small holes to supply ventilation. That container is then placed in a vehicle with a noisy motor, traveling along a bumpy road, with even noisier trucks passing it. When the car stops, you hear dogs barking. Panic. The box, with you still inside, is taken into a building. Your nose is assaulted with the smell of numerous other cats and your arch enemy, dogs. After ten minutes of fear of the sounds and smells of the reception room, the box is transported to another room. The lid opens. Understandably you are reluctant to exit. Your box now seems like the only safe shelter available. An impatient stranger grabs you by the scruff of your neck and places you on a cold stainless steel table. Without a moment's hesitation, that same stranger pushes a cold glass rod into your rectum.

That is how a feline patient feels at the start of an examination. The same emotions would hold true for any species; only the particular circumstances would change. Sensitivity and empathy in the form of a soft voice and gentle petting can greatly reduce an animal's anxiety level. A less apprehensive patient will produce a smoother, more complete physical examination, with few bites and scratches for the veterinarian. Although most veterinarians begin their career with compassion and understanding, their day-to-day routine combined with a pressured time schedule causes some to lose their sensitivity.

Patience is another virtue all veterinarians would love to possess. An animal will always, repeat always, do the worst possible thing at the worst possible time. A cat will purr when you try to listen to its heart with a stethoscope. A dog will blink and then lick your face when you try to examine its eyes. A dog that "marks" every corner of the reception room with urine will certainly be the same dog from whom it becomes next to impossible to obtain a urine sample for testing. Patience and a sense of humor are personality traits required of any veterinarian who is going to enjoy his profession.

A veterinarian needs to be healthy. Handling animals requires dexterity and at least average physical strength. Some clinical tasks, such as delivering calves or horse dentistry, require substantially more than average muscle. Even a minor impairment such as color blindness (so common in males) can affect a veterinarian's ability to assess all visible symptoms and therefore make a correct diagnosis. Another frequently encountered health problem is allergies. Dander from the hair of horses, cats, and dogs and the dust and mold in barns can make life miserable for a veterinarian prone to allergies. This problem is so common that sufferers have banded together to form the Association of Animal Allergic Veterinarians.

A veterinarian needs acute powers of observation. Sight, hearing, touch, and even smell are utilized to establish a diagnosis and evaluate the treatment's effectiveness or the experiment's results. All the laboratory tests in the world cannot replace a good, complete physical examination.

An active veterinarian will eventually get hurt. Regardless of how careful he may be, the danger is always present, particularly when dealing with horses and livestock. A well-placed kick from a horse can fracture bones, cause internal injuries, or even result in death. A sow will fight ferociously to protect her young. Most zoo animals have no desire to be handled by humans (and they let you know it!). When a cow steps on your foot, one quarter of her 1,000 pounds of body weight lands on your big toe. Dog and cat bites can become severely infected, requiring antibiotics or even hospitalization.

Remember, too, that more than 100 diseases are transmissible between animals and humans. While a case of ringworm may be merely annoying, a case of rabies can be fatal. The pregnant female veterinarian is particularly susceptible to zoonoses. Toxoplasmosis is a disease caused by a single-celled protozoan, which is excreted in the feces of infected cats. A pregnant woman who comes in contact with such feces usually does not get sick, but her unborn baby may become infected. The child could be born blind or brain-damaged or could even die. Toxoplasmosis is only one disease against which pregnant veterinarians must take precautions.

Potential dangers to a veterinarian lie not only with the animals and their diseases, but also with the techniques used in medicine. Anesthesia presents one risk. Small amounts of the anesthetic gases that keep a patient asleep are also present in the air in the surgical suite, whether it is a human or veterinary hospital. In the 1960's scientific evidence revealed that exposure to low levels of anesthetic gas caused spontaneous abortion and premature delivery in female surgical nurses and doctors. Later studies demonstrated a high incidence of congenital abnormalities and birth defects in children born not just to women but also men who work in surgery. The release of anesthetic gas into the environment can now be minimized through the use of scavenging devices, which remove the extra gas from the anethesia machine and transport it outside the room.

Another procedure that has potential undesirable side effects is radiology. Even a small amount of radiation can cause severe malformations in fetuses, particularly of the nervous system and the skeletal system. High doses can cause organ damage and sterility in adults. Veterinarians are exposed to a great amount of radiation through the radiographs they take. They minimize their exposure by using properly functioning equipment and protecting their hands and body with lead gloves and aprons. Many lists of radiation safety practices include statements such as, "Never permit pregnant women in the room during diagnostic procedures." The reason is that no level of radiation exposure has been established as being safe during pregnancy. It should be noted that the most susceptible stage of fetal development is the first eight to ten days following conception. Undoubtably, many women veterinarians have exposed their unborn children to radiation before they even knew they were pregnant.

A fact: Animals are dirty. Even the cleanest Puffy, the pampered Pomeranian, is going to have diarrhea at some point in his life. The average dog presented to a veterinary clinic has dirty ears, fleas, and bad breath. Cows are notorious for calving in a muddy creekbed in the dead of winter. Avon has no desire to bottle "fragrance d'pig." Rectal examination of a cow frequently results in a cowpat deposited in your boot. A constant, incessant, and universal battle against odor is waged in every veterinary clinic. If you find it difficult to clean up your dog's mess in the backyard or keep the cat's litter box clean, you should think twice about veterinary medicine as your career choice. If feces, pus, or urine on your hands offends you, choose another profession. (Another casualty of the veterinary profession is dry, chapped hands from constant washing!)

Blood is another familiar companion to the veterinarian. Without a doubt, the veterinarian must have a strong stomach. Surgery, the odor of vomit, infected wounds, and severe injuries demand a cast-iron stomach and nerves of steel. How will you react when a cat is presented who has been cruelly abused, perhaps a broken tail or poked out eyes? Or how about a young calf that died of starvation in winter because its owner didn't realize that it needed supplemental feed? A veterinarian doesn't blink an eye at the dinner table when talk turns to a foal with a weepy, infected wound that has become infested with maggots.

In this recipe for a veterinarian, let's throw in a big dollop of responsibility. Based on the amount of training and the license awarded to an animal doctor, a great deal of respect is accorded to the veterinarian. Accompanying that respect is responsibility. The final decision, the final diagnosis, the final decree comes from the veterinarian.

A willingness to accept responsibility is apparent when a veterinarian agrees to treat a $1,000,000 Thoroughbred racehorse. He is accountable (i.e., liable) for his decisions and treatments. A veterinarian who works for the government is responsible for accurately reporting and controlling livestock diseases that could affect the whole cattle industry. Nationwide, veterinarians are responsible for the health of approximately 115 million cattle, 56 million hogs, and 12 million sheep and lambs, which help make up this country's $40 billion livestock industry. And let's not forget the 8 million horses.

Because veterinarians accept responsibility, they are targets of malpractice lawsuits brought by disgruntled animal owners. Lawsuits against veterinarians are becoming more common. Horses are the most common species involved in litigation. Because of the animal's high cost and the increasing number of suits, equine veterinarians must carry large amounts of liability insurance, often as much as $1,000,000 coverage. Livestock owners can also sue a veterinarian for large amounts. Improper diagnosis or treatment can result in the loss of an expensive animal or even a whole herd.

Pet owners also file suit against a doctor they feel was incompetent or negligent. They seek compensation not only for the cost of the animal but also for the heartbreak and emotional loss the pet's death caused them. Additionally, they can sue for the loss of potential income from the offspring of a purebred breeding bitch or sire. The veterinarian is not responsible for only his own actions. He is also responsible for any incompetence, negligence, or mistakes on the part of his employees.

In a veterinary clinic, a veterinarian is responsible for the health of an animal and also for the safety of the owner. Owners who have been bitten by their own pet or kicked by their own horse at a veterinary clinic have successfully sued the attending veterinarian. According to law, animals in veterinary hospitals are under the care and control of the veterinarian, and it is his responsibility to insure that they hurt no one, not even their owner.

A more subtle form of responsibility is exemplified in treatment of beloved household pets. This liability does not involve lawsuits or malpractice insurance. Rather, it involves the veterinarian's own conscience. Imagine yourself the veterinarian for Mrs. Johnson, an elderly widow whose husband recently passed away. She has always been close to her thirteen-year-old cat "Dolly," but since her spouse's death she has clung to her pet as her main source of companionship. "Dolly" is ill, but her ailment can be corrected with expensive surgery. Mrs. Johnson's social security income is not sufficient to cover several hundred dollars worth of veterinary expenses. How would you handle the situation? Would you recommend "putting Dolly to sleep"? Or, even though you cannot really afford it, would you donate your time and drugs to help "Dolly" and Mrs. Johnson? The owner-pet bond is a very real emotional alliance that intimately involves the pet's doctor.

Yet this compassion must be balanced by a tough spirit. Realize now that as a veterinarian you will not be able to save all the sick and injured animals. In most jobs that deal with animals death is a reality. Some animals are terminally ill and no amount of medical assistance will cure them. Some animals are euthanized because their owners can't afford veterinary services. Other owners can afford it but won't. It is not the veterinarian's right to pass moral judgment on owners. The animal is the possession of the client, and it is his prerogative to decide its fate. Each owner places a different value on his pet, ranging from "family member" status to merely a piece of property bordering on being a nuisance.

A desire to help "all animals" simply isn't realistic. The hard facts of economics are constantly present. Unless you are independently wealthy, your funds will soon be depleted if you try to help every injured animal you find lying beside the road. To repeatedly invest your time and your boss's money in helping a pet of an owner who either can't or won't pay his bill simply results in your losing your job.

Emergency calls, late hours, and missed holidays are well known by every veterinarian in private practice. Are you the type of person who is ready to go at a moment's notice? Or is your personality such that you value, even treasure, your private time? Only you can decide whether the excitement and satisfaction derived from helping a sick animal are worth your interrupted schedule.

A good exercise for the aspiring veterinarian is to picture yourself in the practitioner's position. Imagine yourself enjoying a pleasurable pastime, perhaps viewing a favorite TV program, attending a football game, relaxing with friends, or sitting down to Thanksgiving dinner (worse yet, after Thanksgiving dinner when you're too stuffed to move!). Suddenly the telephone rings; someone needs your veterinary expertise. Don't imagine this predicament just once. Repeat it many times over a period of six months.

Emergencies occur all too frequently, and often with the worst possible timing. A veterinarian in a one-person practice can expect at least one emergency call a night. A dedicated veterinarian must put his personal desires behind his obligations to his career. If, in your imaginary scenario, your find yourself resentful of the situation, then being a veterinarian without access to an animal emergency clinic is definitely not for you. Emergency calls have made more than one veterinarian regret his career choice.

Another important point to remember is that the animals are always accompanied by people. In the small animal veterinary clinic, pets don't find their way to the hospital; owners bring them. The same is true in large animal medicine. Someone has to own the racehorse. Someone has to raise the cattle. In academia, students must be taught. In government and industry, coworkers as well as the general public must be dealt with. The point is that you should not enter veterinary medicine only because you like animals. If you don't like people too, your professional life will be filled with endless frustration.

Before you choose veterinary medicine as a career, be sure your view of the profession is realistic. Recent years have seen an upsurge in the number of burned-out and disillusioned veterinarians. Numerous journal articles and seminars are directed at this problem of overexpectations, disappointments, and unfulfilled dreams. Realize fully, and don't kid yourself, that your salary as a veterinarian will probably never be the equivalent of your potential earnings in other professions. Realize that unless pet medical insurance becomes commonplace, veterinarians will never be able to charge for their services what human medical doctors charge. Realize that a veterinarian will never receive the respect from society that his human counterpart receives. Realize that a forty-hour workweek is an unreasonable expectation for a new graduate.

The veterinary profession is experiencing a generation of veterinarians who are disenchanted with their career. They feel used and abused by their employing veterinarian. Try to remember that your future employer is also trying to survive in a difficult world while carrying a heavy debt burden. In today's society an animal doctor stands a poor chance of receiving generous compensation for his hard work, regardless of his skills in medicine or business management. Are you prepared to accept these facts? Will your future spouse be capable of accepting these facts?

Do you fit the picture of a happy, successful animal doctor? Be sure your character makeup is compatible with that of a veterinarian. Don't make the mistake of finding out that veterinary medicine is not for you after you've completed eight years of college. Career testing is available through most high schools and colleges. Take advantage of it.

Following are the criteria used by the College of Veterinary Medicine at Mississippi State University to subjectively evaluate its applicants. These are the qualities they feel are necessary for the successful completion of the four-year professional program. They are also the qualities they feel a veterinarian should possess. How do you rate?

*Communication skills*
    Fluency of speech
    Poise, bearing, and dress
    Ability to elaborate
    Persuasiveness

*Self-determination*
    Stable work habits
    Pride
    Self-discipline
    Decisiveness
    Completes work
    Self-confidence

*Professionalism*
    Knowledge of veterinary
        profession
    Values toward "life and death"
    Feelings about research on
        animals
    Realistic view of what is
        required of a veterinarian
    Dedication to an ideal

*Adaptability*
 Willingness to learn
 Flexibility
 Resourcefulness

*Maturity*
 Reliability
 Initiative
 Accurate interpretation of
  the actions of others
 Realistic career planning

*Leadership*
 Organizes people and things
 Decision-making ability
 Realistic assessment
  of tasks
 Planful

*Capacity for Service*
 Willingness to help
 Interest in people
 Sympathy and compassion
 Cheerful disposition toward
  work

*Motivation*
 Persistence
 Conscientiousness
 Interest in veterinary
  medicine
 Enthusiasm
 Dedication

*Chapter* **XI**

# What Should You Do Next?

If you still want to pursue a career in veterinary medicine, your next step should be the accumulation of information.

Talk to your educational advisor, and take the courses he or she recommends. Your advisor has access to career testing by which you can find out where your strengths lie. If you're not cut out for medicine, better to find out now than eight years down the road.

Get those grades up and keep them up. Students accepted into veterinary school are A students. Realize that they are your competition. They are the ones who will receive the D.V.M., not the students who put off homework to the last minute. Nor do future veterinarians choose to watch a television movie or sports event when they know they need to "hit the books." Veterinary medicine requires perseverance and dedication to a goal. You might as well start now.

You need to take all the biology courses that are available at your school. The stronger your high school science base, the easier your undergraduate studies. The more advanced science and animal science courses you take in college, the less difficult veterinary college will seem.

Discover what your school and community offer in the way of 4-H and FFA groups. Join up. At least one of their varied activities should spark your interest, and you will undoubtably meet other preveterinary students with whom you can exchange ideas and information.

Develop a financial plan to see you through eight years of college. Are your parents willing to support you through your schooling? Economically, would it be best for you to live at home as long as possible? Will you have to work full time or part time? Perhaps you should consider postponing college for a year or two and working full time to save money to finance your education. How readily available are scholarships and student loans? To make a good financial plan, you should add your tuition and book expenses and your personal living expenses (shelter, food, clothing, transportation, spending money) and compare it to your potential income while in college.

Write to the American Veterinary Medical Association, 930 North Meacham Road, Schaumburg, IL 60196, for information and brochures. Write to the veterinary schools of your choice to find out direct what the requirements and tuition fees are. Keep in touch with them annually, since both will probably change.

Most veterinary colleges hold an annual open house for the public to tour their facilities. This is an excellent opportunity to see a veterinary school as well as view the operation of a large, well-equipped veterinary hospital. It also allows you to talk with veterinary students and find out firsthand what veterinary school is really like. Some colleges arrange private tours of their facilities; check with the school of your choice.

Read the books and references listed at the end of this book. Reading a variety of books will provide a realistic view of the profession. Although James Herriott's *All Creatures Great and Small* series is enjoyable, his works are one-sided in scope and meant to be entertaining rather than informative.

Of utmost importance is gaining actual experience working with animals. Make sure you understand the day-to-day realities of what you are attempting. Even if you have to volunteer your time or work for minimum wage, the experience of a job (preferably two or three) in the field of your choice is priceless.

One obvious place to gain practical experience is at a veterinary clinic. However, finding such a job is not easy. Even though many veterinarians are receptive to helping students, there are many more students than there are jobs (or veterinarians). Establish a rapport with a local veterinarian. If you own pets or livestock, ask questions the next time he treats your animals. Don't act squeamish when he gives your animal an injection or gets feces on his hands. It's part of the job. "Oooo, gross!" is not an appropriate response from a young adult viewing a preserved canine heart infected with heartworms. Ask if he needs help during the summer or on weekends. Fortunately for you, summer and weekends are the veterinarian's busiest times, and he may need an extra hand.

If you manage to obtain an interview, use common sense. Be well groomed and be on time. Use proper grammar. If he offers you a job, expect minimum wage at best. More likely than not, you'll need to volunteer your time. Don't be discouraged if your chores include sweeping floors and cleaning bathrooms. In fact, some young people get their foot in the door by first mowing grass and doing yard work at a clinic. If you persevere, you'll move up the career ladder to disinfecting cages and bathing dogs. The sky's the limit from there!

If your passion is dogs and cats but you cannot find a veterinarian willing to give you experience, try volunteer work at a local humane society or SPCA (Society for the Prevention of Cruelty to Animals). They will probably welcome your unpaid help. Your responsibilities may include cleaning cages and kennels, exercising animals, and assisting the veterinarian (with luck). This can help you learn the various breeds, learn to deal with vicious animals, and learn to cope with death, always a reality in any animal-related business.

Other possibilities for employment include pet stores, grooming shops, and kennels. Although these jobs may not provide direct experience in veterinary medicine, at least you can develop skill in handling animals and make certain that you really want to do it on a daily basis. You may also deal with people, possibly filling out forms, selling pet supplies, collecting money, and items of that nature. This is also good experience. Remember, every veterinarian needs to be able to communicate with people.

Another possibility is to become an entrepreneur by starting your own animal care business. A real need exists in many localities for people willing to "dog sit" while owners are on vacation. Many animals are more content (and therefore their owners are happier) at home rather than in a boarding kennel. You would be responsible for feeding, walking, and brushing the animal two or three times a day. Another business you can start at home is dog bathing/dipping. Many owners would rather pay to have their dog bathed than bother with it themselves. Besides earning money and gaining experience, operating a business at a young age demonstrates initiative. Veterinary schools look favorably on such a résumé.

If working with horses is your forte, experience may be more difficult to acquire. Even volunteer jobs are not easy to find. If you find employment at all, it will probably involve cleaning stalls and, if you're fortunate, grooming horses.

Equine veterinarians, stables, and ranches always need extra help. However, for safety reasons, they require that their helpers know what they're doing. They can't take a chance on your getting hurt. If the veterinarian or the stable seems reluctant for you even to volunteer your time, don't be offended. Like any business, they have their liability to consider. Working around horses provides ample opportunities for injury. Not all horses are as well-mannered as your pet horse. A person can gain "horse sense" only through working with many horses, including some flighty ones.

Mixed animal practitioners seem slightly more receptive to having either volunteer or paid helpers. Some county vets are glad to have someone to talk to while they make their calls. Those many hours alone on the road can be boring.

The initial responsibilities of an assistant to a mixed animal practitioner include "fetching" and "holding." Inevitably, the veterinarian is in the barn or the pasture and needs certain drugs or equipment from his truck. Naturally, his helper is sent to fetch it. Then the veterinarian has both hands full, so the assistant holds the medicine, the rope, the nose tongs, and so on. But the aspiring veterinarian who demonstrates common sense and real desire will eventually get some actual hands-on experience.

Another possibility for urbanites is to look for work on a farm. Some veterinary colleges require their students to have at least minimal exposure to livestock or horses. Perhaps you could work one summer on a farm. Maybe you have a relative or friend who raises livestock. Besides the practical experience, it can be an opportunity for personal growth.

If your interest lies with exotic animals, try to obtain employment at a zoo. Your job may not even include working directly with animals. It may be selling soft drinks at a concession stand. But with initiative, the employment can be quite valuable. Talk to the zoo keepers. This is not the time to be bashful. Ask questions that are well thought out in advance. Plan to stay after work or arrive early to spend time with zoo personnel.

One possibility is taking time off from school to work full time in your area of interest. No requirement says that you have to continue straight through your education. You have a lot of years working as a veterinarian ahead of you. So what if you start wo years later? To really dig down and discover the inner workings of a profession requires time.

Whatever avenue you choose to gain experience, be prepared to work extra hard at it. More than an average amount of drive, enthusiasm, and ambition must be devoted to any project you undertake. If you are not willing to show initiative or to put in extra time and effort now, forget veterinary medicine as a career. It's a demanding profession—on your time, your stamina, and your emotions.

*Chapter* **XII**

# What If You Don't Become a Veterinarian?

Many young people want to work with animals but for one reason or another do not obtain degrees in veterinary medicine. Remember, in the United States only 40 percent of students who apply to veterinary schools are admitted. That translates into over 5,700 applicants for veterinary school every year and more than 3,400 students disappointed. Some students do not get even as far as submitting an application. They are sidetracked by inadequate grades, marriage, lack of motivation, financial difficulties, or family obligations.

Young adults who read this book do so because they think they want to be animal doctors, but it is essential that they keep an open mind to other possibilities. Every preveterinary student needs to have other educational and career paths he can follow as backups to his original plans. Each aspiring veterinarian should have alternative goals so that if his dream of becoming an animal doctor is not attained he has another satisfying career that he can fall back upon. Even a highly motivated person can experience a health, financial, or personal crisis during the years of college that may require him to forgo his primary goal.

*Veterinary Technician*

Such people may find career satisfaction as veterinary technicians. Animal health technology is a branch of animal health care that has evolved in response to an increasing need for qualified personnel to assist veterinarians. They can handle many responsibilities and duties to free the veterinarian for functions for which only he is qualified.

Although anyone working with animals in a medical environment can be called an animal caretaker, a veterinary assistant, or an animal attendant, only graduates of a two-year college-level program are called Animal Health Technicians (AHT). These programs provide formal training in both the scientific and husbandry aspects of animal care. Although informal education can be gained by any lay person working in a veterinary hospital, obtaining a technician's degree confers a broader and deeper view of the job and its responsibilities, as well as allowing the holder to move up the salary ladder faster and higher. Although the vast majority of Animal Health Technicians are women, men are certainly welcome and are becoming more interested in the field.

Some states require that veterinary technicians be licensed, to obtain which educational requirements must be met, an examination must be passed, and a fee paid.

Technicians are employed by both large and small animal practices. Duties may include collecting blood, urine, and fecal specimens, restraining animals, processing radiographs, interacting with clients, monitoring a patient's vital signs, preparing the animal and instruments for surgery, placing catheters, giving medications, and care and feeding of animals. They are well trained in performing laboratory procedures: microscopic fecal checks for worms and other parasites, heartworm tests, blood counts, urinalyses, and blood serum chemistries.

Their duties *do not* include diagnosing, performing surgery, or prescribing drugs. These remain the sole responsibilities of the licensed veterinarian.

Like veterinarians, technicians are supposed to be observant. They are trained to distinguish normal from abnormal, health from disease. In their daily association with the hospitalized animals, they are often in closer contact than the veterinarian is. Many times they are the ones who notice subtle symptoms and changes in the behavior of the animals.

Many technicians also play an integral role in client communications. In the veterinarian's routine, he sees many of the same diseases over and over again. Repeated explanations to the owners can become tedious. The technician can take over some of the responsibilities, informing owners about parasite control, nutrition, and vaccination requirements and answering questions. Many people are slightly intimidated by a doctor and feel less threatened by the technician and therefore freer to ask what they may perceive as "stupid" questions.

Although the majority of technicians work at private veterinary clinics, technicians are also employed by drug companies, hospitals, laboratories, zoos, meat-packing companies, and universities. At hospitals, universities, and private industry, these paraprofessionals deal mainly with rats, monkeys, mice, rabbits, and dogs used in research. Over 25 million such animals are used annually in the U.S. for teaching and research purposes.

Typical annual salaries for technicians range from $8,500 to

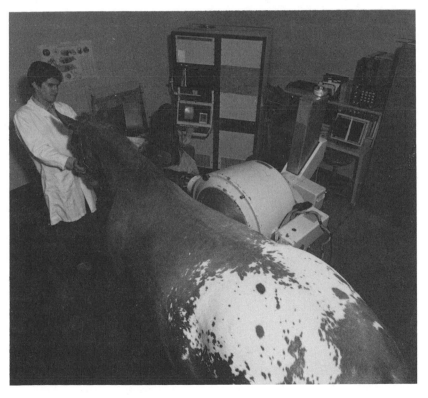

*University of Illinois College of Veterinary Medicine*
A horse is led before a gamma camera during a nuclear medicine scan.

$12,500 for new graduates and $10,000 to $18,000 for experienced technicians. Pay scales may be based on an hourly wage or a straight weekly or monthly salary. Fringe benefits such as health insurance, paid vacation, and profit-sharing and pension plans vary according to the employer. As in any job, the level of compensation depends not only on professional skills but also on qualities such as punctuality, dependability, attitude, appearance, and the ability to communicate and work well with people.

Education involves a two-year college-level program designed to provide both practical and scientific training. The AVMA Committee for Accreditation of Training of Animal Technicians sets the standards for training, evaluates programs, and accredits acceptable programs. Currently 58 schools with programs in animal technology are accredited by the AVMA (see Appendix). New schools are constantly being added. Additional information on veterinary technology may be obtained from the American Veterinary Medical Association, 930 North Meacham Road, Schaumburg, Il 60196. High school counselors should have information on local schools. Most programs require a high school diploma prior to admission.

The curriculum of an animal technology program generally includes the following:

Chemistry
Applied mathematics
Communications skills
Humanities or liberal arts
Biological science
Orientation to the vocation of animal technology
Ethics and jurisprudence in veterinary medicine
Animal husbandry, including restraint, species and breed identification, and sex determination
Principles of veterinary anatomy and physiology
Animal care and management
Biochemistry
Medical terminology
Veterinary office management
Diseases and nursing of companion animals, food production animals, horses, and laboratory animals
Animal nutrition and feeding

Anesthetic nursing and monitoring, including instrumentation
Surgical nursing and assisting including instrumentation
Necropsy techniques
Pharmacology for animal technicians
Radiography, utilizing live animals
Comparative animal hematology
Veterinary urinalysis
Veterinary parasitology
Veterinary clinical biochemistries
Animal microbiology and sanitation
Clinical experience in veterinary practice

The goal of the AHT program is to give students a foundation of practical knowledge upon which to build after employment. There are as many ways to execute procedures in veterinary medicine as there are veterinarians to perform them. The technician is expected to conform to the employer-veterinarian's methods. The final responsibility for a patient, the success or failure of a treatment, rests with the veterinarian. He expects his directions to be followed precisely.

Having a degree in animal health technology allows the employee to be of greater benefit to the business based on broader knowledge. It does not, however, put the technician in a position of being "above" certain duties. Everyone, from the veterinarian to the kennel helper, "scoops poop" in a veterinary facility. Animals are dirty. Dirt, grime, and odor accompany any facility for animals. An employee who refuses to pitch in and help with housekeeping will quickly antagonize his coworkers and cause dissension in the clinic. Unpleasant duties of all animal caretakers include cleaning up manure, urine, blood, and vomit, disinfecting animal areas, sweeping up hair, trimming out fur matted with blood, feces, or pus, and doing battle against fleas and ticks. In the meantime, he tries to keep his own appearance neat and professional looking in the process.

Dr. Michael A. Obenski summed it up in an article in the *DVM Newsmagazine* ("Life in the Trenches Is No Picnic," January 1986, Vol 17, No. 1):

You see, [technicians] have a lot in common with [veterinarians]. Like veterinarians, most technicians and assistants choose their careers out of a desire to work with animals. Unfortunately, both groups soon have to face certain disappointments.

Like learning, for example, that all animals aren't the cute, fluffy friends that we remember from childhood. Some are nasty, smelly, and yes, even dirty.

Both groups must also face the ultimate letdown together. It's something that the guidance counselor never mentioned.

Another reality is the fact that our "cute, fluffy friends" are capable of biting, clawing, nipping, scratching, growling, hissing, kicking, and attacking. Animals, like their owners, are not always rational or well-mannered.

Animal health technology can be a frustrating, yet fulfilling career. One must accept less than desirable hours (usually including weekends and evenings), a great deal of dirt, and a somewhat limited pay scale. However, many technicians truly enjoy playing an integral role in animal health care. They realize that their skills and training enable them to help animals lead healthier, more enjoyable lives. These technicians find the work stimulating, rewarding, and satisfying and wouldn't change professions for anything in the world. Veterinary medicine requires teamwork of the entire professional and paraprofessional staff if the optimum results are to be attained.

*Other Career Options*

Being a veterinary technician is not the only alternative to becoming a veterinarian. Once a young person decides what his desires and abilities are and which species of animals he prefers to work with, many career paths are opened.

One obvious choice is to become a livestock producer. Ranchers can raise cattle, sheep, or goats. Any of these species can be raised for meat. Sheep or goats can be raised for wool or hair. Dairymen are not limited to cows; dairy goats are gaining popularity as very efficient producers of hypoallergenic milk. The main drawback to becoming an animal producer is the large amount of capital required to purchase land, equipment, and animals and the slow return on investment.

Animal caretakers are employed by zoos across the country, but openings are not plentiful. A college background is not required to work in a zoo, but a person with a degree can advance faster and higher. The same is true of marine exhibits such as Sea World.

A love of horses opens many career opportunities. Racehorses require exercisers, groomers, assistant trainers, and trainers. Employees are needed to clean stalls, wrap legs, give medications, and cool down horses after a workout. Pleasure horses require riding instructors and stable owners/managers. Blacksmiths (also known as farriers) are in demand. Blacksmiths must go to school to learn their trade; they must also be strong, since it is backbreaking work.

For people who feel dogs are their specialty, several opportunities exist. Dog groomers not only trim hair but also clean ears, cut toenails, and empty the anal glands located beneath the tail. Groomers are hard workers as well as artistic individuals. Often they must match the dog's haircut to the owner's personality.

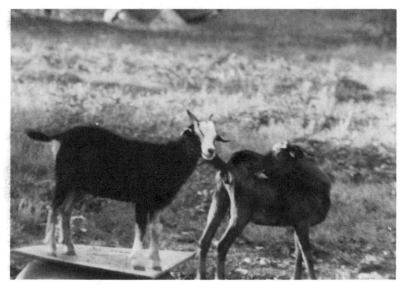

*Norden Laboratories, Inc.*
Goats are rapidly gaining in popularity, both as pets and as a source of hypoallergenic milk.

Show dog and cat handlers are becoming more common. Many people want their animals to win shows but do not want to invest the time that it requires. Professional handlers train the animals and travel across the country to attend shows. Other handlers work with specialty dogs such as guard dogs, police dogs, and dogs for the blind and deaf. Kennel owners get to work around dogs everyday, as do animal shelter employees.

As well as dogs and cats, pet store owners also sell mice, gerbils, guineapigs, hamsters, monkeys, and many varieties of fish and birds. A combination of talent in photography and the ability to inspire trust in animals can result in a career as a pet photographer. A special rapport with animals is required of a Hollywood or circus animal trainer. Many high school and college animal science departments have actual herds of animals from which students learn. Advisors are needed for young people involved in 4-H and FFA. County agricultural extension agents are involved in a similar service geared toward livestock producers.

# Appendix

*COLLEGES OF VETERINARY MEDICINE
IN THE UNITED STATES AND CANADA*

Auburn University
College of Veterinary Medicine
Auburn, AL 36849

Tuskegee University
School of Veterinary Medicine
Tuskegee, AL 36088

University of California
School of Veterinary Medicine
Davis, CA 95616

Colorado State University
College of Veterinary Medicine
Ft. Collins, CO 80523

University of Florida
College of Veterinary Medicine
Gainesville, FL 32610

University of Georgia
College of Veterinary Medicine
Athens, GA 30602

University of Illinois
College of Veterinary Medicine
Urbana, IL 61801

Purdue University
School of Veterinary Medicine
West Lafayette, IN 47907

Iowa State University
College of Veterinary Medicine
Ames, IA 50011

Kansas State University
College of Veterinary Medicine
Manhattan, KS 66506

Louisiana State University
School of Veterinary Medicine
Baton Rouge, LA 70803

Tufts University
School of Veterinary Medicine
North Grafton, MA 01536

Michigan State University
College of Veterinary Medicine
East Lansing, MI 48824–1316

University of Minnesota
College of Veterinary Medicine
St. Paul, MN 55108

Mississippi State University
College of Veterinary Medicine
Mississippi State, MS 39762

University of Missouri
College of Veterinary Medicine
Columbia, MO 65211

Cornell University
New York State College of Veterinary Medicine
Ithaca, NY 14853

North Carolina State University
School of Veterinary Medicine
Raleigh, NC 27606

Ohio State University
College of Veterinary Medicine
Columbus, OH 43210

Oklahoma State University
College of Veterinary Medicine
Stillwater, OK 74078

Oregon State University
College of Veterinary Medicine
Corvallis, OR 97331

University of Pennsylvania
School of Veterinary Medicine
Philadelphia, PA 19104

University of Tennessee
College of Veterinary Medicine
Knoxville, TN 37901

Texas A & M University
Texas Veterinary Medical Center
College Station, TX 77843

Virginia Tech & University of Maryland
Virginia–Maryland Regional College of Veterinary Medicine
Blacksburg, VA 24061

Washington State University
College of Veterinary Medicine
Pullman, WA 99164

University of Wisconsin–Madison
School of Veterinary Medicine
Madison, WI 53706

Ontario Veterinary College
University of Guelph
Guelph, Ontario, Canada N1G 2W1

University of Prince Edward Island
Altantic Veterinary College
Charlottetown, P.E.I, Canada CIA 4P3

University of Montreal
Faculty of Veterinary Medicine
Saint Hyacinthe
Quebec, Ontario, Canada J2S 7C6

University of Saskatchewan
Western College of Veterinary Medicine
Saskatoon, Saskatchewan, Canada S7N 0W0

## ACCREDITED PROGRAMS IN ANIMAL TECHNOLOGY

**Alabama**
Snead State Junior College
Animal Hospital Technology Program
Boaz, AL 35957

**California**
Cosumnes River College
Animal Health Technology Program
8401 Center Parkway
Sacramento, CA 95823

Hartnell College
Animal Health Technician Program
156 Homestead Avenue
Salinas, CA 93901

Los Angeles Pierce College
Animal Health Technology Program
6201 Winnetka Avenue
Woodland Hills, CA 91371

Mt. San Antonio College
Animal Health Technology Program
1100 North Grand Avenue
Walnut, CA 91789

San Diego Mesa College
Animal Health Technology Program
7250 Mesa College Drive
San Diego, Ca 92111

Yuba College
Animal Health Technician Program
Beale Road 2088 North
Marysville, CA 95901

**Colorado**
Colorado Montain College
Animal Health Technology Program
Spring Valley Campus
3000 C. Road 114
Glenwood Springs, CO 81601

Bel-Rea Institute of Animal Technology
1681 South Dayton Street
Denver, CO 80231

**Connecticut**
Quinnipiac College
Laboratory Animal Technology Program
Mt. Carmel Avenue
Hamden, CT 06518

**Florida**
St. Petersburg Junior College
Veterinary Technology Program
Box 13489
St. Petersburg, FL 33733

**Georgia**
Abraham Baldwin Agriculture College
Veterinary Technology Program
Box 8, ABAC Station
Tifton, GA 31793

Fort Valley State College
Veterinary Technology Program
Fort Valley, GA 31030

**Illinois**
Parkland College
Veterinary Technology Program
2400 West Bradley Avenue
Champaign, IL 61821

**Indiana**
Purdue University
School of Veterinary Medicine
Veterinary Technology Program
West Lafayette, IN 47907

**Kansas**
Colby Community College
Animal Technology Program
1255 South Range
Colby, KS 67701

**Kentucky**
Morehead State University
Veterinary Technology Program
Box 995
Morehead, KY 40351

**Louisiana**
Northwestern State University of Louisiana
Veterinary Technology Program
Department of Agricultural Sciences
Natchitoches, LA 71457

**Maine**
University of Maine
Animal Medical Technology Program
Department of Animal and Veterinary Sciences
Orono, ME 04473

**Maryland**
Essex Community College
Animal Science Technology Program
7201 Rossville Boulevard
Baltimore, MD 21237

Essex Community College
Walter Reed Army Institute of Research
Animal Science Technology Program
7201 Rossville Boulevard
Baltimore, MD 21237

**Massachusetts**
Newberry Junior College
Animal Health Technician Program
100 Summer Street
Boston, MA 01746

Becker Junior College
Veterinary Assistant Program
1003 Old Main Street
Leicester, MA 01524

**Michigan**
Macomb Community College
Veterinary Technician Program
Center Campus
Mt. Clemens, MI 48044

Michigan State University
College of Veterinary Medicine
Veterinary Technology Program
East Lansing, MI 48823

Wayne Community College
Veterinary Technology Program
c/o Wayne State University
Department of Laboratory Animal Resources
540 East Canfield Street
Detroit, MI 48201

**Minnesota**
Medical Institute of Minnesota
Veterinary Technician Program
2309 Nicollet Aveneue
Minneapolis, MN 55404

University of Minnesota
Animal Health Technology Program
Waseca, MN 56093

**Missouri**
Maple Woods Community College
Animal Health Technology Program
2601 NW Barry Road
Kansas City, MO 64156

Northeast Missouri State University
Animal Health Technology Program
Kirksville, MO 63501

Jefferson College
Animal Health Technology Program
Hillsboro, MO 63050

**Nebraska**
University of Nebraska
School of Technical Agriculture
Veterinary Technology Program
Curtis, NE 69025

Omaha College of Health Careers
Animal Technician Program
1052 Park Avenue
Omaha, NE 68105

**New Jersey**
Camden County College
Animal Science Technology Program
P.O. Box 200
Blackwood, NJ 08012

**New York**
State University of New York
Agricultural and Technical College
Agriculture and Life Sciences
Veterinary Science Technology Program
Canton, NY 13617

La Guardia Community College
The City University of New York
Animal Health Technology Program
31–10 Thomson Avenue
Long Island City, NY 11101

State University of New York
Agricultural and Technical College
Veterinary Science Technology Program
Delhi, NY 13753

**North Carolina**
Central Carolina Technical College
Veterinary Medical Technology Program
1105 Kelly Drive
Sanford, NC 27330

**North Dakota**
North Dakota State University
Animal Health Technician Program
Department of Veterinary Science
Fargo, ND 58102

**Ohio**
Columbus Technical Institute
Animal Health Technology
550 East Spring Street
Columbus, OH 43215

Raymond Walters College
Animal Health Technology Program
University of Cincinnati
Cincinnati, OH 45221

**Oklahoma**
Murray State College
Veterinary Assistant Technology Program
Tishomingo, OK 73460

**Pennsylvania**
Harcum Junior College
Animal Health Technician Program
Bryn Mawr, PA 19010

Median School of Allied Health Careers
Animal Health Technology Program
121–9th Street
Pittsburgh, PA 15222

Wilson College
Veterinary Medical Technology Program
Chambersburg, PA 17201

**South Carolina**
Tri-County Technical College
Veterinary Technology Program
P.O. Box 587
Pendleton, SC 29670

**South Dakota**
National College
Animal Health Care Program
P.O. Box 302
Rapid City, SD 57709

**Tennessee**
Columbia State Community College
Animal Health Technology Program
Columbia, TN 38401

**Texas**
Cedar Valley College
Animal Medical Technology Program
3030 North Dallas Avenue
Lancaster, TX 75134

Sul Ross State University
Range Animal Science Department
Animal Health Technician Program
Alpine, TX 79830

Texas State Technical Institute
Animal Technology Program
James Connally Campus
Waco, TX 76705

**Utah**
Brigham Young University
Animal Health Technology Program
Provo, UT 84602

**Virginia**
Blue Ridge Community College
Animal Technology Program
Box 80
Weyers Cave, VA 24486

Northern Virginia Community College
Animal Science Technology Program
Loudoun Campus
1000 Harry Flood Byrd Highway
Sterling, VA 22170

**Washington**
Fort Steilacoom Community College
Animal Technology Program
9401 Farwest Drive SW
Tacoma, WA 98498

**West Virginia**
Fairmont State College
Veterinary Assistant Technology Program
Fairmont, WV 26554

**Wisconsin**
Madison Area Technical College
Animal Technician Program
211 North Carroll Street
Madison, WI 53703

**Wyoming**
Eastern Wyoming College
Animal Health Technology Program
3200 West C Street
Torrington, WY 82240

# Bibliography

Berger, Melvin. *Animal Hospital*. Toronto: Fitzhenry & Whiteside Limited, 1973.

Bridges, William. *Zoo Doctor*. New York: William Morrow & Company, 1957.

Camuti, Louis J. *All My Patients Are Under the Bed*, New York: Simon & Schuster, 1980.

Compton, Grant. *What Does a Veterinarian Do?* New York: Dodd, Mead & Co., 1964.

Cutris, Patricia. *Animal Doctors: What It's Like to Be a Veterinarian and How to Become One*. New York: Delacorte Press, 1977.

Haddock, Sally. *The Making of a Woman Veterinarian*. New York: Simon & Schuster, 1985.

Hart, Susanne. *Too Short a Day: A Woman Veterinarian in Africa*. New York: Taplinger Publishing Co., 1966.

————. *Listen to the Wild: A Woman Vet's Further African Adventures*. New York: Taplinger Publishing Co., 1972.

Herriott, James. *All Creatures Great and Small*. New York: St. Martin's Press, 1972.

————. *All Things Bright and Beautiful*. New York: Bantam, 1974.

————. *All Things Wise and Wonderful*. New York: Bantam, 1977.

————. *The Lord God Made Them All*. New York: St. Martin's Press, 1981.

————. *The Best of James Herriott*. New York: St. Martin's Press, 1982.

Hughes, John. *The Animals Came In*. New York: Taplinger Publishing Co., 1971.

May, Charles Paul. *Veterinarians and Their Patients*. New York: Thomas Nelson & Sons, 1964.

McCoy, Joseph J. *The World of the Veterinarian*. New York: Lothrop, Lee & Shepard, 1954.

McDonnell, Virginia. *Dixie Cline Animal Doctor*. Camden: Thomas Nelson and Sons, 1966.

Morrisson, James W., and Wignall, Robert F. *VAT Veterinary College Admissions: A Comprehensive Guide*. New York: Arco Publishing Co, 1985.

Perry, John. *Veterinarians and What They Do*. New York: Franklin Watts, 1964.

Price, Mary Lee. *Ms. Veterinarian*. Philadelphia: Westminster Press, 1977.

Schwabe, Calvin W. *Veterinary Medicine and Human Health*. Baltimore: Williams and Williams Co., 1969.

Shay, Arthur. *What Happens at a Veterinary Hospital*. Chicago: Rilly & Lee Books, 1972.

Swope, Robert E. *Opportunities in Veterinary Medicine*. Skokie, IL: VGM Career Horizons, 1978.

"Today's Veterinarian," pamphlet available from the American Veterinary Medical Association, 930 North Meacham Road, Schaumburg, IL 60172.

*Veterinary Medicine: A Career of Choices*, sponsored by the American Association of Veterinary Medical Colleges. Order from Office of Student Affairs & Admissions, New York State College of Veterinary Medicine, C-117 Shurman Hall, Cornell University, Ithaca, NY 14853.

*Veterinary Medicine Schools Admissions Requirements in the United States and Canada*. Bethesda, MD: Betz Publishing Co, Inc.

Vine, Louis L. *Dogs Are My Patients*. Jericho, New York: Exposition Press, 1971.

Whitney, Leon. *Animal Doctor: The Satisfaction of a Career in Veterinary Medicine*. New York: McKay, 1973.

Wright, John W. *The American Almanac of Jobs and Salaries*. New York: Avon Books, The Hearst Corp., 1984.

Yates, Elizabeth. *Is There a Doctor in the Barn?* New York: E.P. Dutton & Co., 1966.

Young, Wesley A., and Miklowitz, Gloria. *The Zoo Was My World*. New York: E.P. Dutton & Co., 1969.

# Index